Je

The Ultimate Weight Watchers Points Guide.

Weight Watchers Points for Thousands of Items Which Were Calculated Using the Nutrition Values.

Are you losing weight with Weight Watchers?

Millions of people have used the Weight Watchers diet. The unique way that it works means that you can eat anything you like, so long as you don't go over your daily allocation of points.

Keeping track of the thousands of food items that area available can be hard work, but with this great new book, **The Ultimate Weight Watchers Points Guide: Weight Watchers Points for Thousands of Items Which Were Calculated Using the Nutrition Values,** you will have instant information on:

- The points system
- Nutritional values of foods
- WW points for 1500 products
- Easy to see what foods are within your daily budget

This revolutionary and simple-to-use system has seen millions lose weight and keep it off. Thanks to the points system you can see exactly what you can and cannot afford to eat. In addition to that you can also get more of a daily allowance, depending on the exercise you take, so it encourages you to be more active too.

And with **The Ultimate Weight Watchers Points Guide** you will have another friend to help you keep track of your weight loss and make sure you stay on course to shed those unwanted pounds.

Get your copy today! Losing weight has never been easier.

What is Weight Watchers?

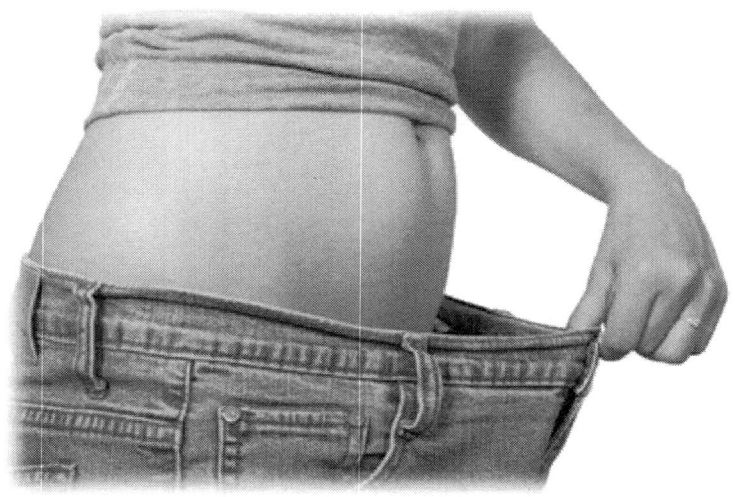

Weight Watchers International was founded in 1963 by Jean Nidetch. It is now an International company operating in over 30 countries across the world. It is the world's leading organization in weight loss management helping millions of people to lose weight since its inception over 50 years ago. Jean Nidetch was an overweight housewife who had unsuccessfully tried many other diet programs.

In 1961, she was introduced to a food sponsored by the New York City Board of Health, through the successful implementation of this diet she lost 20 pounds. She was amazed at her success and wanted to share her story. She formed a support group with her overweight friends and then regular weekly classes. The popularity of these meetups grew and grew; she initially started in just her apartment in Queens, New York.

However, she quickly outgrew her apartment and moved to professional business meeting locations. The phenomenon then rapidly expanded across America and then across the world. Now an internationally known brand, it was owned by the Heinz group from 1978 to 1999. Now boasting thousands if not millions of success stories across the world, it continues to soar with Oprah Winfrey on its panel of board members, who also owns 10% of the company. It has become a worldwide success. It all began with Jean Nidetch trying to lose weight.

The principle of Weight Watchers

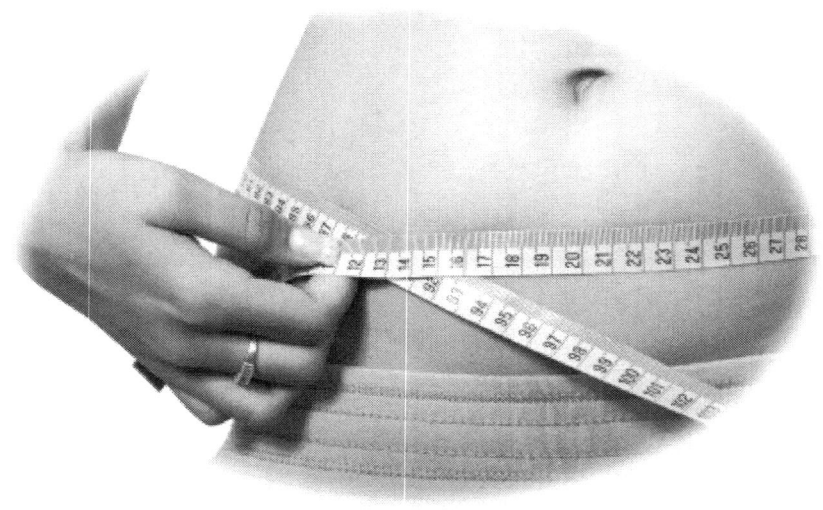

The principle of Weight Watchers is based on nutritional science and a program geared towards sustainable success. You are taught which foods and what food types are healthiest for you. This allows you to make healthier food decisions and no food is banned from the Weight Watchers program. This means it works alongside other diets and personal lifestyle choices. It also means that you don't feel limited or constricted in adopting this diet.

The goal is to lose weight through calorie reduction in a sustainable fashion through healthy eating. It also encourages the implementation of an exercise program and offers a local support group. You are invited to track your use and movements through activity tracker gadgets like the Fitbit. This will allow you to analyze what exercise you are doing and how it will work alongside your diet. The third principle is the support group where you will meet like-minded local people with this same aspirations has you.

You will also be guided by a success coach who has been on the same journey, has you? This is a vital part of Weight Watchers, and statistically, the more somebody attends the local meetings, the higher the likelihood of their success. It gives you the opportunity to tap into the wealth of knowledge available in the network and having a support group enhances your possibility of really succeeding long term.

Therefore, Weight Watchers operates on three key principles; healthy eating, a regular exercise program and a support group. There is also an online option where you don't attend meetings, but you have the opportunity to be part of an online community and network.

The program is very simple to follow and access to help readily available in the form of coaches, resources or the online or offline community. Firstly, you will have a confidential weigh in and set your ideal weight goal based upon your body mass index. If you are successful in this goal, you then begin a maintenance period for six weeks. This phase is to establish stability in your weight, and if successfully implemented you will become a lifetime member.

It's success factors are based upon a coach who has achieved success through the Weight Watchers program and a like-minded network which offers support, accountability, ideas and inspiration. This combined with the wealth of knowledge and tools online like the app, recipe ideas, expert chat facility, fitness videos and support network makes you realize why it is the market leader in weight loss management.

The Weight Watchers points system

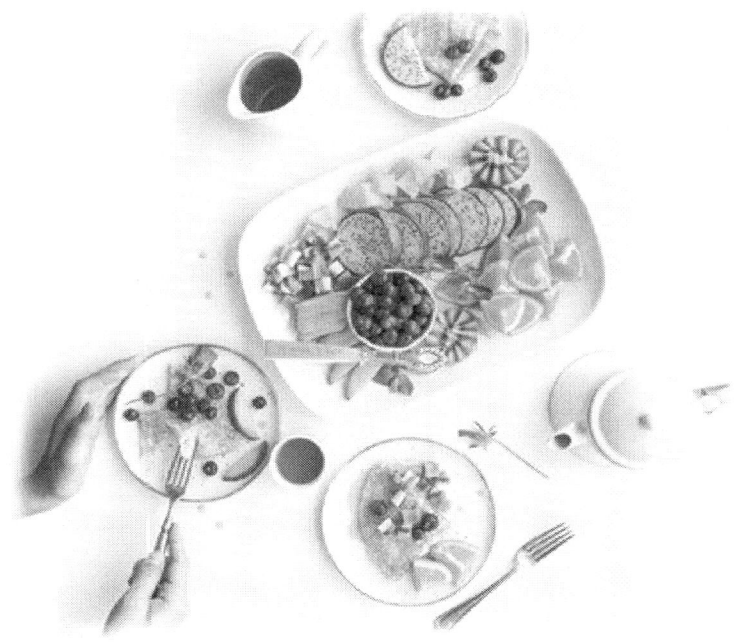

The Weight Watchers points system is simple and straightforward. All foods are turned into points based upon their nutritional value. You are allocated a budget of points based upon your goal and target. You must not exceed your daily target of points, and if you don't, you will lose weight. The basic premise is that calories are the baseline for how many points a particular food is worth. This means that sugar and saturated fat will increase points and healthier foods will keep you on target. The result will be that you will eat more fruit, vegetables and lean protein but less sugar and saturated fat to keep you on target. You can track all of this easily online or through an app. You can carry your points over day to day but critically not week to week.

Weight Watchers has successfully adapted to the online age by creating tools and resources. You can track your points online, read and post in forums and chatrooms, discover healthy tips and advice. If you have a certain amount of points remaining it will even give you recipe suggestions. It also creates charts and graphs based on your exercise and eating trends. This allows you to stay on track and collect valuable data on your performance. Another great feature is almost all major restaurants are logged on to its system enabling you to easily identify what it best for you to eat when you go out for a meal with friends or family.

The secret of success

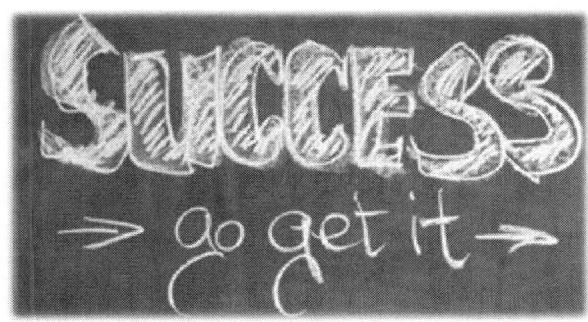

The secret of success in the Weight Watchers diet is that it simply works if you use it correctly.

- It encourages simplicity of diet while still giving you free reign over what you can eat.
- It is not restrictive but built in a way which is supportive of your goals.
- It encourages you to eat in moderation and regularly.
- Its success is firmly rooted in the support group and community system.

The key to losing weight is following its simple formula and plugging into its local and online community and group. Here you will find the leading edge of weight management techniques and advice supported by like minded, local people from your community.

Weight Watchers Points

„In the table below, find your current weight. Next to your weight range is the range of Weight Watchers points you should be eating in a single day. For example, if you currently weigh 230lbs, you'd be in the 225-249lb range. Your Weight Watchers point range would be 26-31 points. In any given day, you should aim to eat at least 26 points, but no more than 31 points. It's important to eat at least the minimum number of points in your range. Otherwise, you risk your body going into 'starvation mode' and not losing any weight at all.

Target Weight Watchers Points Ranges

Weight	Points
Less than 150	18-23
150-174	20-25
175-199	22-27
200-224	24-29
225-249	26-31
250-274	28-33
275-299	29-34
300-324	30-35
325-349	31-36
More than 350	32-37

Below that table is a comprehensive list of foods and their Weight Watchers point values. Use that table to keep track of how many points you eat in a day. If you're looking for something that isn't on the list but you have the nutritional information, you can do a little math and get an idea of the point value. 50 calories = 1 point, 6 grams of fat = 1 point, and you can subtract 1 point for every 4 grams of fiber. So the calculation for something that is 250 calories, 12 grams of fat, and 4 grams of fiber would be: $(250/50) + (12/6) - (4/4) = (5) + (2) - (1) = 6$ Weight Watchers points."*

*Source: http://www.quiddity.cc/rachel/diet/wwfoods.html

Beans & Legumes

#	Name	Amount	Points
1	Beans, baked	1/2 cup	5
2	Beans, baked, canned	1/2 cup (4 oz.)	2
3	Beans, baked, deli	1/2 cup (4 oz.)	3
4	Beans, baked, fast food	1 serving	4
5	Beans, baked, vegetarian, canned	1/2 cup (4 oz.)	2
6	Beans, Black, and rice mix (prepared according to package directions)	1 cup	4
7	Beans, Black, cooked	1/2 cup	2
8	Beans, Black, refried	1/2 cup	1
9	Beans, Black, refried, canned, low-fat or fat-free	1/2 cup	1
10	Beans, Black, uncooked	1 pound	31
11	Beans, Cannellini, cooked	1/2 cup	1
12	Beans, Garbanzo, cooked	1/2 cup	2
13	Beans, Garbanzo, uncooked	1 pound	35
14	Beans, Green, cooked	1 cup	0
15	Beans, Kidney, cooked	1/2 cup	1
16	Beans, Kidney, uncooked	1 pound	30
17	Beans, Lima, cooked	1/2 cup	1
18	Beans, Lima, uncooked	1 pound	30

#	Name	Amount	Points
19	Beans, Navy, cooked	1/2 cup	2
20	Beans, Navy, uncooked	1 pound	30
21	Beans, Pinto, cooked	1/2 cup	2
22	Beans, Pinto, uncooked	1 pound	30
23	Beans, Red, and rice	1 cup	5
24	Beans, Red, and rice mix (prepared according to package directions)	1 cup	5
25	Beans, Refried,	1/2 cup	3
26	Beans, Refried, canned	1/2 cup	2
27	Beans, Refried, fat-free, canned	1/2 cup	2
28	Beans, Refried, with sausage, canned	1/2 cup	5
29	Beans, Wax, cooked	1 cup	0
30	Beans, White, cooked	1/2 cup	2
31	Beans, White, uncooked	1 pound	30
32	Chickpeas, dry	1/3 cup or 2 oz. cooked or 3/4 oz. uncooked	1
33	Daiquiri	1 (3 fl. oz.)	3
34	Daiquiri mix	1/2 cup (4 fl. oz.) mix	3

#	Name	Amount	Points
35	Lentils, dry	1/3 cup or 2 oz. cooked or 3/4 oz. uncooked	1
36	Soybeans, dry	1/3 cup or 2 oz. cooked or 3/4 oz. uncooked	1
37	Sprouts, alfalfa	1 cup (1 oz.)	0
38	Sprouts, bean	1 cup (4 oz.)	0

Beverages (non alcohol)

#	Name	Amount	Points
1	Apple Cider	1/2 cup (4 fl. oz.)	1
2	Apple Juice	1/2 cup (4 fl. oz.)	1
3	Beer, non-alcoholic	1 can or bottle (12 fl. oz.)	1
4	Coffee mix, flavored, sugar-free (prepared according to package directions)	1 cup (8 fl. oz.) prepared	1

#	Name	Amount	Points
5	Coffee mix, flavored, with sugar (prepared according to package directions)	1 cup (8 fl. oz.) prepared	1
6	Cranberry juice cocktail, low-calorie	1 cup (8 fl. oz.)	1
7	Cranberry juice cocktail, regular	1/2 cup (4 fl. oz.)	1
8	Eggnog, reduced-calorie, without liquor	1/2 cup (4 fl. oz.)	3
9	Eggnog, store-bought, without liquor	1/2 cup (4 fl. oz.)	5
10	Eggnog, without liquor	1/2 cup (4 fl. oz.)	4
11	Fruit cocktail, unsweetened, canned	1 cup (9 oz.)	2
12	Fruit drink mix, powdered	8 fl. oz. prepared	2
13	Fruit juice, combined, any type	1/2 cup (4 fl. oz.)	1
14	Grape juice (carbonated or non-carbonated)	1/2 cup (4 fl. oz.)	1
15	Grapefruit juice, any type	1/2 cup (4 fl. oz.)	1
16	Hot chocolate, homemade, with whipped topping	1 cup (8 fl. oz.)	7
17	Hot chocolate, homemade, without whipped topping	1 cup (8 fl. oz.)	6

#	Name	Amount	Points
18	Ice cream soda	1 (12 fl. oz.)	8
19	Irish coffee	1 (6 fl. oz. with 2 tbsp. whipped cream)	4
20	Latte, made with fat-free milk	1 small (8 fl. oz.)	2
21	Latte, made with fat-free milk	1 tall (12 fl. oz.)	2
22	Latte, made with fat-free milk	1 grande (16 fl. oz.)	3
23	Latte, made with low-fat milk	1 small (8 fl. oz.)	3
24	Latte, made with low-fat milk	1 tall (12 fl. oz.)	4
25	Latte, made with low-fat milk	1 grande (16 fl. oz.)	4
26	Latte, made with whole milk	1 small (8 fl. oz.)	3
27	Latte, made with whole milk	1 tall (12 fl. oz.)	5
28	Latte, made with whole milk	1 grande (16 fl. oz.)	6
29	Lemonade	1 cup (8 fl. oz.)	2

Beverages (alcohol)

#	Name	Amount	Points
1	Beer, regular	1 can or bottle (12 fl. oz.)	3
2	Beer, light	1 can or bottle (12 fl. oz.)	2
3	Black Russian	1 (3 fl. oz.)	5
4	Bloody Mary	1 (5 fl. oz.)	2
5	Brandy	1 1/2 fl. oz.	2
6	Brandy Alexander	1 (3 fl. oz.)	8
7	Champagne	1 small glass or 1/2 cup (4 fl. oz.)	2
8	Cognac	1 1/2 fl. oz.	2
9	Eggnog, with liquor	1/2 cup (4 fl. oz.)	4
10	Gin	1 jigger (1 1/2 fl. oz.)	2
11	Gin and tonic	1 (6 fl. oz.)	4
12	Gin gimlet	1 (2 1/2 fl. oz.)	3
13	Liqueurs, any type	1 jigger (1 1/2 fl. oz.)	4
14	Liquor (gin, rum, scotch, tequila, vodka, whiskey)	1 jigger (1 1/2 fl. oz.)	2
15	Tom Collins	1 (6 fl. oz.)	3
16	Vodka	1 jigger (1 1/2 fl. oz.)	2
17	Vodka gimlet	1 (2 1/2 fl. oz.)	3

#	Name	Amount	Points
18	Whiskey	1 jigger (1 1/2 fl. oz.)	2
19	Whiskey sour	1 (3 fl. oz.)	3
20	Wine cooler	1 (8 fl. oz.)	3
21	Wine spritzer	1 (8 fl. oz.)	2
22	Wine, dessert, dry	2 fl. oz.	1
23	Wine, dessert, sweet	2 fl. oz.	2
24	Wine, light	4 fl. oz.	1
25	Wine, regular, dry	1 small glass or 1/2 cup (4 fl. oz.)	2

Breads & Crackers

#	Name	Amount	Points
1	Animal crackers	13(1 oz.)	3
2	Bagel, any type	1 small or 1/2 large (2 oz.)	3
3	Banana Bread	1 slice (5" x 3/4")	5
4	Banana Bread, with nuts	1 slice (5" x 3/4")	5
5	Boston brown bread	1 slice (3 3/4" x 1/2") or 1 1/2 oz.	2
6	Bread crumbs, dried	3 tbsp (3/4 oz.)	1
7	Bread crumbs, dried	1 cup	9
8	Bread crumbs, seasoned	3 tbsp.	2
9	Bread, any type (white, wheat, rye, Italian, French, pumpernickel)	1 slice (1 oz.)	2
10	Bread, cocktail(party-style), any type	2 slices (3/4 oz.)	1
11	Bread, high-fiber, (3 grams or more dietary fiber per slice)	1 slice (1 oz.)	1
12	Bread, Indian(Navajo)fry	1 (5" diameter)	6
13	Bread, reduced-calorie, any type	2 slices (1 1/2 oz.)	1
14	Breadstick, soft	1 (1 1/4 oz.)	2
15	Breadsticks	2 long (7 1/2" x 1/2") or 4 short (5" x 1/2")	1

23

#	Name	Amount	Points
16	Croissant, chocolate-filled	1 (5" long) or 1 3/4 oz.	6
17	Croissant, plain	1 (5" long) or 1 3/4 oz.	5
18	Date nut bread	1 slice (5" x 1/2")	5
19	Fadge	1 cup	3
20	Flatbreads	3/4 oz.	1
21	Focaccia	1 piece (10" diameter)	25
22	Focaccia bread, any type, store-bought	2 oz.	3
23	Garlic bread, frozen	1 piece	4
24	Graham cracker crumbs	2 tbsp.	1
25	Graham crackers	2 (2 1/2" squares) or 1/2 oz.	1
26	Graham crackers, chocolate-covered	2 (1/2 oz.)	2
27	Graham crackers, mini, any variety	3/4 oz.	2
28	Hamburger bun,	1	3
29	Hamburger bun, light,	1	2
30	Hamburger bun, reduced-calorie	1	1
31	Irish soda bread	1/12 of 8" round loaf or 3 1/2 oz.	5
32	Lavash	1/4 of 10" cracker or 2 1/4 oz.	6

Cereal

#	Name	Amount	Points
1	Cereal, Cold, any type (other than those listed below)	1 cup	2
2	Cereal, Cold, Bran Flakes	3/4 cup	1
3	Cereal, Cold, fortified	1 cup	2
4	Cereal, Cold, frosted	1 cup	3
5	Cereal, Cold, granola	1/2 cup	4
6	Cereal, Cold, granola, homemade	1/2 cup	6
7	Cereal, Cold, granola, low-fat	1/2 cup	3
8	Cereal, Cold, nuggets	1/2 cup	3
9	Cereal, Cold, puffed	1 cup	1
10	Cereal, Cold, raisin bran	3/4 cup	1
11	Cereal, Cold, shredded wheat	1 biscuit	1
12	Cereal, Cold, whole-grain	1 cup	2
13	Cereal, Hot, cream of rice	1 cup	2
14	Cereal, Hot, cream of wheat	1 cup	2
15	Cereal, Hot, farina, cooked	1 cup	2
16	Cereal, Hot, farina, uncooked	1/4 cup	3
17	Cereal, Hot, grits	1 cup	3
18	Cereal, Hot, grits, uncooked	1/4 cup	3
19	Cereal, Hot, oatmeal, cooked	1 cup	3

#	Name	Amount	Points
20	Cereal, Hot, oatmeal, flavored, cooked	1 packet	3
21	Cereal, Hot, oatmeal, uncooked	1 cup	6
22	Hominy grits	1 cup cooked (9 oz.) or 1 1/2 oz. uncooked	2
23	Hominy, whole	1 cup cooked	2
24	Kasha (buckwheat groats)	1 cup cooked or 2 oz. uncooked	3
25	Millet	1/3 cup cooked or 3/4 oz. uncooked	1
26	Quinoa	2 tbsp. dry (3/4 oz.)	1
27	Wheat germ	3 tbsp. (3/4 oz.)	1
28	Wheat germ	1 tsp.	0

Cheese

#	Name	Amount	Points
1	Cheese ball, store-bought	2 tbsp. (1 oz.)	3
2	Cheese, cheddar, soup, canned(made with low-fat or skim milk)	1 cup	4
3	Cheese, cheddar, soup, canned(made with whole milk)	1 cup	5
4	Cheese, cottage, 1% or nonfat, with fruit	1/3 cup	2
5	Cheese, cottage, 1%, 2%, or nonfat	1/3 cup (2 3/4 oz.)	1
6	Cheese, cottage, regular or 4%	1/3 (2 1/2 oz.)	2
7	Cheese, low-fat, hard or semisoft	1 slice, 1 (1") cube, 3 tbsp. shredded, 2 tbsp. grated or 3/4 oz.	2
8	Cheese, Neufchatel	1 tbsp. (1/2 oz.)	1
9	Cheese, nonfat, hard or semisoft	1 slice, 1 (1") cube, 3 tbsp. shredded, 2 tbsp. grated, or 3/4 oz.	1
10	Cheese, pot	1/3 cup	1

#	Name	Amount	Points
11	Cheese, regular, hard or semisoft	1 slice, 1 (1") cube, 3 tbsp. shredded, 2 tbsp. grated, or 3/4 oz.	2
12	Cheese, ricotta, nonfat	1/3 cup	1
13	Cheese, ricotta, part-skim	1/3 cup	3
14	Cheese, ricotta, whole milk	1/3 cup	4
15	Fromage frais (soft cheese with fruit)	3 1/2 oz.	3
16	Soy cheese, nonfat	1 slice, 1 (1") cube, 3 tbsp. shredded, 2 tbsp.grated or 3/4 oz.	1
17	Soy cheese, regular	1 slice, 1 (1") cube, 3 tbsp. shredded, 2 tbsp. grated or 3/4 oz.	2

Condiments, Dressings, Marinades & Spreads

#	Name	Amount	Points
1	Arrowroot	1 tsp.	0
2	Bacon bits, imitation	1 tsp	0
3	Baking powder or soda	1 tsp.	0
4	Bean dip, fat-free	1/2 cup (4 oz.)	1
5	Beets, pickled	1/2 cup	1
6	Chutney	1 tbsp.	1
7	Cocktail sauce	1/4 cup	1
8	Concentrated yeast extract	1 tsp.	0
9	Cream, clotted (English double devon cream)	2 tbsp.	4
10	Cream, light (coffee/table cream)	2 tbsp (1fl. oz.)	2
11	Cream, medium	2 tbsp. (1 fl. oz.)	2
12	Cream, whipped, homemade (no sugar added)	1/4 cup	3
13	Cream, whipping, heavy or light	2 tbsp. (1 fl. oz.)	3
14	Dip, any type	2 tbsp.	2
15	Dip, Artichoke, baked	1/4 cup	6
16	Dip, Spinach	1/4 cup	5
17	Eggs, substitute, fat-free	1/4 cup	1
18	Etouffee mix	2 tbsp. mix	1

Condiments, Dressings, Marinades & Spreads

#	Name	Amount	Points
19	Filo dough, frozen	1 oz. (about 1 1/2 sheets)	2
20	Fructose	1 tbsp	1
21	Giardeniera (vegetable medley, without olives, packed in vinegar)	1 cup	0
22	Guacamole	1/4 cup	2
23	Guacamole, store-bought	1/4 cup (2 oz.)	2
24	Gumbo base (seasoning mix)	1 1/2 tbsp. (1/2 oz.)	1
25	Hazelnut and chocolate spread	1 tbsp. (1/2 oz.)	2
26	Herring, pickled	1/2 cup	2
27	Honey	1 tbsp.	1
28	Honey	1 cup	20
29	Hummus, any type	1/4 cup	3
30	Hummus, store-bought	1/4 cup	2
31	Hush puppy mix	1/4 cup mix (1 oz.)	3
32	Ketchup	1/4 cup	1
33	Phyllo dough, frozen	1 oz. (about 1 1/2 sheets)	2
34	Sweet and sour mix	1/2 cup (4 fl. oz.) mix	2

Dairy Products

#	Name	Amount	Points
1	Buttermilk baking mix	3 tbsp.	2
2	Buttermilk, dry	1/4 cup powder	2
3	Buttermilk, nonfat, 1%, 1.5%, or 2%	1 cup (8 fl. oz.)	2
4	Cream cheese, light or whipped	2 tbsp. (1 oz.)	1
5	Cream cheese, nonfat	4 tbsp. (2 oz.)	1
6	Cream cheese, regular	1 tbsp. (1/2 oz.)	1
7	Cream cheese, tofu	2 tbsp. (1 oz.)	2
8	Creamer, nondairy	2 tbsp liquid (1 fl. oz.)	1
9	Creamer, nondairy	1 tbsp. powder	1
10	Creamer, nonfat, flavored	2 tbsp. liquid (1 fl. oz.)	1
11	Dairy shake, reduced-calorie	1 packet	2
12	Yogurt and cucumber salad	1/4 cup	1
13	Yogurt bar, chocolate-covered	1	5
14	Yogurt drink	1 cup (8 fl. oz.)	5
15	Yogurt, low-fat, sweetened with sugar, flavored(vanilla, lemon, coffee)	1 cup	4
16	Yogurt, low-fat, sweetened with sugar, fruit-flavored	1 cup	5

#	Name	Amount	Points
17	Yogurt, plain	1 cup	4
18	Yogurt-covered pretzels	7 (8 oz.)	3
19	Yogurt-covered raisins	2 z.	3

Desserts & Sweet Treats

#	Name	Amount	Points
1	Ambrosia	1/2 cup	2
2	Angel Food Cake	1/16 of 10" tube or 2 oz.	2
3	Apple Brown Betty	1 cup	5
4	Apple crisp	3/4 cup	8
5	Apple, baked	1 large	7
6	Apple, candied	1 large	10
7	Apple, caramel	1 large	9
8	Apple, dried	1/4 cup(3/4 oz.)	1
9	Baba au rhum	1	8
10	Bakalava, store-bought	1 piece (1 1/2 oz.)	5

#	Name	Amount	Points
11	Baked Alaska	1 piece (2" wedge)	5
12	Baklava	1 piece (2" square)	5
13	Banana Split	1 serving (3 scoops ice cream, 1 banana, 3 tbsp. syrup, and 1/2 cup whipped cream)	19
14	Bananas Foster	1 serving (2 scoops ice cream, 1/2 banana and 1/3 cup sauce	16
15	Beef Wellington	1 slice (3 1/2" x 2 1/2" x 1 1/2") or 5 oz.	12
16	Beignet	1 (2" diameter)	2
17	Beignet, from mix (prepared according to pkg. directions)	1	3
18	Brioche	1 (1 oz.)	3
19	Brownie	1 (2" square)	5
20	Brownie, fat-free, store-bought	1 (1 1/2 oz.)	2
21	Brownie, low-fat, store-bought	1 (1 1/2 oz.)	3
22	Cake mix, light, without icing	1/12 of prepared 9" cake	4

#	Name	Amount	Points
23	Cake, cupcake, creme-filled, store-bought	1	4
24	Cake, fat-free, store-bought	1 slice (3 1/2 oz.)	4
25	Cake, snack, creme-filled, store-bought	2(2 1/4 oz.)	6
26	Cake, sugar-free, store-bought	1 slice (2 1/2 oz.)	5
27	Cake, with icing	1/12 of 9" layer cake or 3" square	12
28	Cake, with icing, store-bought	1 slice (3 oz.)	7
29	Candy corn	1 oz.	2
30	Candy, Caramels	1 oz.	2
31	Candy, Chocolate, any type	1 oz. (2 assorted pieces, 1/2 candy bar, or 2 tbsp. chips)	4
32	Candy, Gumdrops	1 oz.	2
33	Candy, Hard	1 oz.	2
34	Candy, Jellybeans	10 (1 oz.)	2
35	Candy, Licorice	1 rope (43" long)	1

#	Name	Amount	Points
36	Candy, Licorice	1 oz.	2
37	Candy, mint, chocolate-covered	1 (2 1/4" diameter)	3
38	Candy, sesame	1 piece (2" x 1")	2
39	Candy, taffy	1 piece (1/2 oz.)	1
40	Cannoli	1 (3 1/2" long)	9
41	Caramels	1 oz.	3
42	Carrot cake, with cream cheese icing	1/12 of 9" cake or 3" square	16
43	Cereal bar, fat-free	1 (1 1/2 oz.)	2
44	Cereal bar, fruit filled	1 (1 1/3 oz.)	3
45	Cheesecake	1/16 of 9" cake	7
46	Cheesecake, fast food	1 serving	7
47	Cheesecake, with fruit topping	1/16 of 9" cake	7
48	Cheesecake, with fruit topping, fast food	1 serving	8
49	Cherries, chocolate-covered	2 (1 oz.)	2
50	Chiffon pie	1/8 of 9" one-crust pie	8
51	Chocolate mousse	1 cup	11

#	Name	Amount	Points
52	Chocolate, any type	2 assorted pieces, 1/2 candy bar, 2 tbsp. chips or 1 oz.	3
53	Cinnamon bun	1 (3" diameter) or 2 oz.	5
54	Coconut-custard pie	1/8 of 9" one crust pie	
55	Coffee cake	3" square or 1/12 of 9" tube	6
56	Coffee cake, fat-free, store-bought	1 serving (2 oz.)	3
57	Coffee cake, store-bought	1 serving (2 oz.)	5
58	Cotton Candy	1 (1 1/2 oz.)	3
59	Crab cakes	2 (each 2 1/4 oz. or 3" round)	7
60	Cream pie, with fruit	1/8 of 9" one-crust pie	9
61	Cream pie, with or without fruit, frozen	1 slice (4 3/4 oz.) of one-crust pie	10
62	Cream pie, without fruit	1/8 of 9" one-crust pie	9
63	Cream puff	1 (2 oz.)	9
64	Creme caramel	1 cup	5
65	Crepes	2 (6" diameter)	5

#	Name	Amount	Points
66	Crepes suzette	2	12
67	Crepes, chicken	2	16
68	Crepes, seafood	2	13
69	Cruller	1 small or 1/2 large (1 oz.)	3
70	Crumpet	1	2
71	Cupcake, with icing, creme-filled, store-bought	1 (1 1/2 oz.)	3
72	Cupcake, with icing, unfilled	1 (3" diameter)	5
73	Custard	1 cup	6
74	Custard pie	1/8 of 9" one-crust pie	7
75	Danish, fast food	1	8
76	Danish, store-bought	1 (2 1/4 oz.)	6
77	Doughnut holes, yeast, glazed	2	3
78	Doughnut, cake-type, with icing	1 (3" diameter)	7
79	Doughnut, holes, yeast, glazed	2	3
80	Doughnuts, any type, store bought	1 (2 oz.)	5
81	Doughnuts, cake-type	1 (3" diameter)	6

#	Name	Amount	Points
82	Doughnuts, cake-type, sugared or glazed	1 (3 " diameter)	6
83	Doughnuts, mini, chocolate-covered, store-bought	3-4 doughnuts (2 oz.)	7
84	Doughnuts, mini, powdered sugar-covered, store bought	3-4 doughnuts (2 oz.)	6
85	Doughnuts, with creme filling	1 (3 1/2"x 2 1/2" oval)	8
86	Doughnuts, yeast, plain or glazed	1 (3 " diameter)	6
87	Doughnuts, yeast, with jelly filling	1 (3 1/2" x 2 1/2" oval)	7
88	Eclair	1 (4" long)	9
89	Empandas	2 (3" diameter)	3
90	Flan	3/4 cup	8
91	Franks in blankets, frozen	6 (3 oz.)	9
92	Fried ice cream	1 scoop (1/2 cup)	9
93	Frosting, store-bought, regular or reduced-fat	2 tbsp (1 oz.)	3
94	Fruit compote	1/2 cup	4
95	Fruit ice	1 scoop (1/2 cup)	3

#	Name	Amount	Points
96	Fruit juice bar, frozen	1 (2 1/2 oz.)	1
97	Fruit juice bars, no sugar added, frozen	2 (each 2 oz.)	1
98	Fruit juice cup, frozen	1 (6 1/2 oz.)	3
99	Fruit pie filling, canned	1/3 cup (3 oz.)	2
100	Fruit pie filling, light, canned	1/3 cup (3 oz.)	1
101	Fruit pie, individual, store-bought	1 (4 1/2 oz.)	10
102	Fruit salad	1 cup (9 oz.)	2
103	Fruitcake	1 slice (2 1/2" x 1 3/4" x 1/2") or 2 oz.	4
104	Fruit-flavored pieces	1 package	2
105	Fruit-flavored rolls	1 large	1
106	Fruit-flavored rolls	1 small	1
107	Fudge, plain	1 piece (1" x 2") or 1 oz.	3
108	Funnel cake	1/2 (8" diameter)	12
109	Gingerbread	3" square	6
110	Green tea ice cream	1 scoop (1/2 cup)	4
111	Gumdrops	8 (1 oz.)	3

#	Name	Amount	Points
112	Halvah	1 piece (2" x 1 3/4" x 1")	5
113	Halvah, store-bought	1 1/2 oz.	6
114	Haroset	1 cup	4
115	Honey bun, glazed	1 (4' x 3" oval)	6
116	Honey cake	1 slice (5" x 3" x 1")	7
117	Honey roll	1	5
118	Ice cream bar, chocolate-covered	1 (3 fl. oz.)	5
119	Ice cream bar, chocolate-covered, with crisp rice, no sugar added	1 (1 1/2 oz.)	3
120	Ice cream bar, chocolate-covered, with crisp rice, sweetened with sugar	1 (2 oz.)	5
121	Ice cream cone, plain or sugar	1 small	1
122	Ice cream sandwich	1	4
123	Ice cream sandwich, reduced-calorie	1	4

#	Name	Amount	Points
124	Ice cream sundae	1 scoop (1/2 cup) ice cream with syrup, nuts, and whipped topping	8
125	Ice cream sundae cone	1 (3 1/2 oz.)	8
126	Ice cream, fat-free, no sugar added	1 scoop (1/2 cup)	2
127	Ice cream, fat-free, sweetened with sugar	1 scoop (1/2 cup)	2
128	Ice cream, fried	1 scoop (1/2 cup)	11
129	Ice cream, light, no sugar added	1 scoop (1/2 cup)	2
130	Ice cream, light, sweetened with sugar	1 scoop (1/2 cup)	3
131	Ice cream, premium	1 scoop (1/2 cup)	7
132	Ice cream, regular	1 scoop (1/2 cup)	4
133	Italian Ice, resturant prepared	1/2 cup	1
134	Kataifi	1 piece (2" long)	5
135	Key Lime pie	1/8 of 9" one-crust pie	12

#	Name	Amount	Points
136	Kheer	1/2 cup	5
137	Lollipop	1 (1 oz.)	2
138	Marshmallows	2 medium (1/2 oz.)	1
139	Marzipan	1 oz.	3
140	Meringue pie, any type	1/8 of 9" pie	9
141	Meringue pie, any type, frozen	1 slice (5 oz.)	7
142	Mince pie, frozen	1 slice (4 1/2 oz.) of two-crust pie	7
143	Mincemeat pie, with meat	1/8 of 9" two-crust pie	14
144	Mincemeat pie, without meat	1/8 of 9" two-crust pie	14
145	Mincemeat, store-bought	1/4 cup (2 1/2 oz.)	3
146	Mint, chocolate-covered	1 (2 1/2" diameter)	3
147	Molasses, light or blackstrap	1 tbsp.	1
148	Muffin, any type (other than bran)	1 large (3" diameter) or 4 oz.	6
149	Muffin, any type (other than bran), store-bought	1 large (4 oz.)	10
150	Muffin, any type (other than bran), store-bought	2 mini (each 1 oz.)	6

#	Name	Amount	Points
151	Muffin, any type, fast food	1	6
152	Muffin, bran	1 large (3" diameter) or 4 oz.	5
153	Muffin, bran, store-bought	1 large (4 oz.)	9
154	Muffin, breakfast (egg and cheese with sausage, ham, or canadian bacon on English muffin), frozen	1 (4 1/2 oz.)	7
155	Muffin, Englixh, any type	1 (2 oz.)	2
156	Muffin, fat-free	1 small, 1/2 large, or 2 oz.	2
157	Napoleon	1 (4 1/2" x 2" x 1 1/2")	13
158	Nectar, any type	1/2 cup (4 fl. oz.)	1
159	Nectarine	1 (4 oz.)	1
160	Pancake and sausage on a stick	1 (2 oz.)	5
161	Pancake, any type, homemade, frozen, or made from mix	1 (4" diameter)	2
162	Pancakes, Chinese	3	2
163	Pancakes, fast food	3, without margarine and syrup	6

#	Name	Amount	Points
164	Pancakes, mini, frozen, without syrup	6 (2 1/4 oz.)	3
165	Panettone	1/12 of 9" tube or 1 1/2 oz.	6
166	Peach melba	1 scoop (1/2 cup) ice cream with 2 peach halves and raspberry sauce	8
167	Pecan pie	1/8 or 9" one-crust pie	11
168	Pecan pie, frozen	1 slice (4 1/2 oz.) of one-crust pie	10
169	Petit fours	2 (each 1 3/4" x 1 1/2" x 1")	3
170	Pie crust, any type	1/8 of 9" one-crust pie	5
171	Pie crust, any type	1/8 of 9" two-crust pie	7
172	Pie crust, any type, refrigerated or frozen	1/8 of 9" one-crust pie	2
173	Pierogies, cabbage	4 (each 3 1/2")	12
174	Pierogies, cheese	4 (each 3 1/2")	12
175	Pierogies, meat	4 (each 3 1/2")	12
176	Pierogies, potato	4 (each 3 1/2")	12

#	Name	Amount	Points
177	Pierogies, potato and cheese	3 (4 oz.)	4
178	Pierogies, potato and cheese or onion, low-fat, frozen	3 (4 oz.)	4
179	Pot pie, any type, fast food	1	17
180	Pot pie, beef, chicken, or turkey, frozen	1 (7 oz.)	10
181	Pot stickers (filled won tons), pork or vegetable, frozen	1 (1 1/2 oz.) or 2 (each 3/4 oz.)	2
182	Potato pancake mix	3 tbsp. mix (3/4 oz.)	1
183	Potato pancake, frozen	1 (2 oz.)	1
184	Pound cake	1 slice (5" x 3" x 1")	9
185	Pound cake, store-bought	1 slice (2 1/2 oz.)	6
186	Profiterole	1 small (1 oz.)	2
187	Puff pastry dough, frozen	2 oz.	6
188	Pumpkin pie	1/8 of 9" one-crust pie	8
189	Pumpkin pie, frozen	1 slice (5 oz.) of one-crust pie	6
190	Rhubarb pie	1/8 oof 9" two-crust pie	11
191	Rice cakes, other than plain	1 (1/2 oz.)	1
192	Rice cakes, plain	2 (3/4 oz.) or 6 mini	1

#	Name	Amount	Points
193	Rugalach	1 piece (2 1/2" x 1 1/4"), 1 oz.	3
194	Sachertort	1/16 of 9" cake	8
195	Sesame candy	1 piece (2" x 1")	2
196	Shepard's pie	1 cup	9
197	Sherbet	1 scoop (1/2 cup)	3
198	Shortcakes, store-bought	2 (each 1 oz.)	4
199	Sopaipillas	2 (each 4" x 3")	2
200	Sorbet	1 scoop (1/2 cup)	2
201	Spanakpita	3" square	9
202	Spanakpita, frozen	2 pieces (each 1 oz.)	4
203	Sponge cake	1/12 of 9" tube	4
204	Spumoni	1 scoop (1/2 cup)	6
205	Squab	1 oz. cooked	1
206	Strawberry shortcake	1/12 of 9" cake or 1 filled individual shortcake	7
207	Strudel, any type	1 piece (5 1/2" x 2")	8
208	Sugar, any type	1 tbsp.	1
209	Sweet potato pie	1/8 of 9" one-crust pie	8

46

#	Name	Amount	Points
210	Sweet roll	1 (3" diameter) or 2 oz.	5
211	Sweet roll, pecan-swirl, store-bought	2 small (each 1 oz.)	5
212	Sweet roll, store-bought	1 (2 oz.)	5
213	Taffy	1 oz.	3
214	Tarte aux fruits	1/8 of 9" tart	7
215	Tarte aux fruits	4" fruit	10
216	Tirami su	1 piece (2 1/4" square)	10
217	Toaster pastry, low-fat	1 (1 3/4 oz.)	4
218	Toaster pastry, regular, plain or with icing	1 (1 3/4 oz.)	4
219	Tortoni	1 serving	7
220	Trifle	1 cup	5
221	Turnover, fruit, any type	1 (3" x 1 1/2")	4
222	Turnover, fruit, any type, fast food	1	7
223	Tyropitas, frozen	2 (each 1 oz.)	4
224	Zabaglione	1/2 cup	4
225	Zeppole	1 (4" diameter)	5
226	Zuppa Inglese	1/16 of 10" cake	7

Eggs

#	Name	Amount	Points
1	Egg white	1/2	0
2	Egg whites	3	1
3	Omelet,cheese,2-egg	1	8
4	Omelet,ham and cheese,2-egg	1	9
5	Omelet,herb or plain,2-egg	1	6
6	Omelet,vegetable,2-egg	1	7

Entrees & Side Dishes

#	Name	Amount	Points
1	Arroz con pollo	3 oz. chicken with 1 1/2 cups rice	13
2	Artichoke, hearts, cooked	1 cup (6 oz.)	1
3	Artichokes, cooked	1 medium	0
4	Artichokes, marinated	1/2 cup	3
5	Baba ganosh	1/4 cup	3
6	Baba ganosh, store-bought	1/4 cup	3
7	Bacon, lettuce, and tomato sandwich	1	12
8	Bagel pizzas, mini, any type, frozen	4 (3 oz.)	4
9	Barbeque beef sandwich, frozen, microwave	1 (5 oz.)	9
10	Bean and Lentil stew (Dal maharani)	1 cup	6
11	Beans and Franks	1 cup	11
12	Beef goulash	1 cup	8
13	Beef stew	1 cup	5
14	Beef stew, canned	1 cup	6
15	Beef stew, frozen	1 cup	3
16	Beef Stroganoff with noodles	2 cups (1 cup stroganoff with 1 cup noodles)	15
17	Beef, Roast, open-face sandwich with gravy	1	9

#	Name	Amount	Points
18	Beef, roast, sandwich, fast-food	1	8
19	Bialy	1 (3 oz.)	5
20	Blanquette of veal	2 cups	13
21	Broccoli rice casserole	1 cup	5
22	Broccoli stir-fry	1 cup	3
23	Brunswick stew	1 1/2 cups	5
24	Bruschetta	1 slice	3
25	Bubble and squeak	1 cup	3
26	Buffalo wings, cooked	3	9
27	Buffalo wings, frozen(prepared without fat)	3	4
28	Bulgur, cooked	1 cup	2
29	Burrito, bean	1 large (8" long)	8
30	Burrito, bean	1 small (6" long)	5
31	Burrito, bean and cheese, reduced-fat, store-bought	1 (5 1/2 oz.)	5
32	Burrito, bean and cheese, store-bought	1 (5 oz.)	6
33	Burrito, bean, fast food	1	6

#	Name	Amount	Points
34	Burrito, beef and bean, store-bought	1 (5 oz.)	8
35	Burrito, beef or chicken and cheese, reduced-fat, store-bought	1 small or 1/2 large (4 oz.)	4
36	Burrito, beef, with cheese	1 large (8" long)	8
37	Burrito, beef, with cheese	1 small (6" long)	5
38	Burrito, breakfast(egg, cheese, &bacon, ham or sausage), store-bought	1 (3 1/2 oz.)	5
39	Burrito, chicken, store-bought	1 (5 oz.)	6
40	Burrito, chicken, with cheese	1 large (8" long)	7
41	Burrito, chicken, with cheese	1 small (6" long)	5
42	Cabbage, stuffed	2 rolls (3" x 2 1/2")	6
43	Caesar salad	3 cups	7
44	Calamari, fried	1/2 cup	11
45	Calzone	1 (5 1/4" x 6") or 7 oz.	12
46	Caponata	1 cup	2

#	Name	Amount	Points
47	Caponate(eggplant appetizer), store-bought	1/4 cup (2 oz.)	2
48	Carne asada	4 oz.	10
49	Cassoulet	1 cup	11
50	Cellophane noodles	1 cup cooked or 1 1/2 oz. uncooked	3
51	Ceviche	1/2 cup	2
52	Chalupa (pork and bean dish)	1 cup	6
53	Cheese sandwich, grilled, resturant-style	1	13
54	Cheese sandwich, with bacon, grilled	1	16
55	Cheeseburger on bun, double, fast food	1	13
56	Cheeseburger on bun, double, with bacon, fast food	1	15
57	Cheeseburger on bun, fast food	1 large	15
58	Cheeseburger on bun, fast-food	1 small	8

#	Name	Amount	Points
59	Cheeseburger on bun, without mayonnaise, lettuce, and tomato	1	10
60	Cheeseburger, microwave, frozen	9	
61	Cheeseburger, witth bacon, microwave, frozen	1 (5 oz.)	11
62	Chef's salad, without dressing	4 cups	8
63	Chef's salad, witthout dressing, fast food	1	4
64	Chicken a la king	3/4 cup	10
65	Chicken and meatball fricassee	2 cups	9
66	Chicken caccitore	5 oz.	13
67	Chicken cordon bleu	1 piece (5 1/2 oz.)	12
68	Chicken cordon bleu, frozen	1 piece (6 3/4 oz.)	10
69	Chicken creole, without rice	1 1/2 cups	9
70	Chicken Kiev	1 serving (4" x 8")	18
71	Chicken Kiev, frozen	1 (6 oz.)	13
72	Chicken parmigiana	1 serving (5 1/2 oz.)	13

#	Name	Amount	Points
73	Chicken parmigiana patty, frozen	1 patty with sauce (5 oz.)	6
74	Chicken salad	1/2 cup	6
75	Chicken salad sandwich	1	10
76	Chicken salad, Oriental	2 cups	7
77	Chicken salad, store-bought	1/2 cup (3 1/2 oz.)	5
78	Chicken sandwich, fried, fast food	1	12
79	Chicken sandwich, grilled, fast food	1	9
80	Chicken sandwich, grilled, frozen	1 (4 1/2 oz.)	6
81	Chicken stew, canned	1 cup (8 1/2 oz.)	4
82	Chicken tetrazzini	1 1/2 cups	9
83	Chicken with cashews	1 cup	11
84	Chicken with dumplings	3 oz. chicken with 2 dumplings	7
85	Chili con carne, with beans	1 cup	7
86	Chili con carne, without beans	1 cup	8

#	Name	Amount	Points
87	Chili con queso	1/4 cup	3
88	Chili con queso, canned	1/4 cup (2 oz.)	2
89	Chili con queso, frozen	1/4 cup (2 oz.)	5
90	Chili dog on a roll	1	10
91	Chili mac, canned	1 cup (8 oz.)	5
92	Chili rellenos	2	16
93	Chimichanga, beef	1 (3" x 3 1/2")	11
94	Chimichanga, beef or chicken, with beans, frozen	1 (6 1/2 oz.)	8
95	Chimichanga, chicken	1 (3" x 3 1/2")	10
96	Chinese vegetables, with beef or pork	1 cup	8
97	Chinese vegetables, with chicken	1 cup	7
98	Chinese vegetables, with shrimp or tofu	1 cup	5
99	Cholent	1 1/2 cups	5

#	Name	Amount	Points
100	Chow mein noodles, homemade or packaged	1/2 cup	3
101	Chow mein noodles, with chicken or shrimp	1 cup	6
102	Chow mein, beef, chicken, or pork, canned	1 cup	1
103	Chow mein, noodles, with beef or pork	1 cup	7
104	Cioppino	1 1/2 cups	6
105	Club sandwich	1	16
106	Cobb salad (without dressing)	3 cups	12
107	Cobbler, fruit, any type	1 cup	7
108	Cobbler, fruit, frozen	4 1/2 oz.	6
109	Coleslaw	1/2 cup	3
110	Coleslaw, fast food	1 serving	5
111	Coleslaw, store-bought	1/2 cup (3 1/2 oz.)	4
112	Coq au vin	2 cups (7 oz.)	13
113	Couscous in a cup	1 (2 oz. dry)	4

#	Name	Amount	Points
114	Couscous, (semolina)	1 cup cooked (6 oz.) or 2 oz. uncooked	3
115	Creole, chicken, without rice	1 1/2 cups	9
116	Creole, fish, without rice	1 1/2 cups	6
117	Creole, shrimp, store-bought	1 cup (9 1/2 oz.)	5
118	Croque Monsieur	1	8
119	Dhansak	1 cup	6
120	Dolma	4	4
121	Dolma, store-bought	4 (3 1/2 oz.)	3
122	Donair	4 oz. meat witth onion, tomato and 2 tbsp. sauce	14
123	Doro wat	1 cup	7
124	Dumplings, beef or pork, fried	4	11
125	Dumplings, beef or pork, steamed	4	6
126	Dumplings, chicken, fried	4	9
127	Dumplings, chicken, steamed	4	4

#	Name	Amount	Points
128	Dumplings, shrimp, fried	4	9
129	Dumplings, shrimp, steamed	4	4
130	Egg foo yung, Beef	1 (3" diameter)	4
131	Egg foo yung, Chicken	1 (3" diameter)	4
132	Egg foo yung, Pork	1 (3" diameter)	5
133	Egg foo yung, Shrimp	1 (3" diameter)	4
134	Egg roll wrapper	1 (1/2 oz.)	1
135	Egg roll, Beef	1 (4 1/2" long)	5
136	Egg roll, Chicken	1 (4 1/2" long)	4
137	Egg roll, Chicken, store-bought	1 (3 oz.)	3
138	Egg roll, Pork	1 (4 1/2" long)	5
139	Egg roll, Pork, store-bought	1 (3 oz.)	3
140	Egg roll, Shrimp	1 (4 1/2" long)	4
141	Egg roll, Shrimp, store-bought	1 (3 oz.)	3
142	Egg roll, Vegetable	1 (3 oz.)	3
143	Egg salad	1/2 cup	7
144	Egg salad sandwich	1	10
145	Eggplant Parmigiana, frozen	5 oz.	4

#	Name	Amount	Points
146	Eggplant Parmigiana, with sauce	1 serving (3" x 4"), with 1/2 cup Italian tomato sauce	13
147	Eggplant Parmigiana, without sauce	1 serving (3" x 4")	11
148	Eggs Benedict	2 English muffin halves with 2 eggs and 1/4 cup hollandaise sauce	16
149	Eggs, Deviled	2 stuffed halves	4
150	Eggs, Fried	1 large	2
151	Eggs, scrambled	2 2 or 1/2 cup	5
152	Eggs, scrambled	1/4 cup.>2/td>	
153	Eggs, scrambled	2 (scrambled with 2 tsp. fat)	6
154	Eggs, scrambled, fast food	1 serving	4
155	Enchilada meal, beef, cheese, or chicken, frozen (2 enchiladas, beans, & rice)	1 (11 1/2 oz.)	7

59

#	Name	Amount	Points
156	Enchilada, beef, cheese, or chicken, store-bought	1 (4 1/2 oz.)	4
157	Enchiladas, beef, cheese or pork	2	12
158	Enchiladas, chicken	2	11
159	Escargots	9 snails with 2 tbsp. butter	9
160	Etouffee, crawfish or shrimp, store-bought	1 cup (9 oz.)	8
161	Fajita kit, beef or chicken, frozen (prepared according to package directions)	2 (7 1/2 oz.)	5
162	Fajitas, Beef	2	11
163	Fajitas, Chicken	2	8
164	Fajitas, Pork	2	13
165	Fajitas, Shrimp	2	8
166	Falafel in pita	1 large pita with 4 falafel patties (each 2" diameter or 1/2 oz.)	13
167	Falafel patties	4 (each 2" diameter or 1/2 oz.)	10

#	Name	Amount	Points
168	Falafel patties, from mix (prepared according to package directions)	2	4
169	Fish and brewis	1 cup	13
170	Fish and cheese sandwich, fried, fast food	1	13
171	Fish and chips	5 oz. fish fillet with 20 chips (french-fries)	16
172	Fish fillet, battered, frozen (prepared without fat)	1 small (3 oz.)	5
173	Fish fillet, grilled, with garlic butter, frozen	1 (3 3/4 oz.)	3
174	Fish fillet, grilled, with lemon pepper, frozen	1 (3 3/4 oz.)	3
175	Fish fillet, sandwich, frozen	1 (4 1/2 oz.)	8
176	Fish fillets, breaded, frozen (prepared without fat)	2 (3 3/4 oz.)	7
177	Fish fillets, light, breaded, frozen (prepared without fat)	3 1/4	3

#	Name	Amount	Points
178	Fish portions, breaded or battered, prepared from minced fish, frozen (prepared without fat)	3 oz.	5
179	Fish sticks, breaded, frozen	4	4
180	Fish Veronique	6 oz.	11
181	Flauta, Beef	1 (6" x 1 1/4")	12
182	Flauta, Chicken	1 (6" x 1 1/4")	10
183	Flauta, Pork	1 (6" x 1 1/4")	11
184	Garlic bread	1 slice (1 oz.)	4
185	Gefilte fish	1 piece (2 1/2 oz.)	2
186	General Tso's chicken	1 cup	15
187	Gnocchi, any type	1 cup	7
188	Gnocchi, cheese	1 cup	13
189	Gnocchi, potato	1 cup	4
190	Gnocchi, spinach	1 cup	9
191	Greek salad, with dressing	3 cups	8
192	Gyro	1 (6")	12
193	Ham, glazed, with pineapple	4 oz. ham with 1/2 pineapple slice	6

#	Name	Amount	Points
194	Hamburger, dinner in a box	1 cup prepared	7
195	Herring in cream sauce, store-bought	1/4 cup (2 oz.)	3
196	Herring in wine sauce, store-bought	1/2 cup (2 oz.)	2
197	Herring salad	1/4 cup (2 oz.)	3
198	Huevos rancheros	2 eggs on 2 tortillas	14
199	Hush puppies	2	4
200	Hush puppies, frozen (prepared without fat	3 (2 oz.)	2
201	Instant breakfast	1 envelope prepared with 1 cup reduced-fat(2%) milk	5
202	Instant breakfast	1 envelope prepared with 1 cup fat-free milk	4
203	Instant breakfast	1 envelope prepared with 1 cup whole milk	6
204	Irish brown stew	1 cup	7
205	Jambalaya mix	1/4 cup (1 1/2 oz.)	3
206	Jambalaya, chicken, with rice	1 1/2 cups	9

#	Name	Amount	Points
207	Jambalaya, fish, with rice	1 1/2 cups	7
208	Kabobs, beef, chicken, or lamb	2 skewers	8
209	Kabobs, fish	2 skewers	6
210	Kasha varnishkes	1 cup	4
211	Kibbe, baked	3 (1 1/2" squares)	3
212	Kibbe, uncooked	1/2 cup	4
213	Kim Chee (Korean-style pickled vegetables)	1 cup (4 oz.)	0
214	Kishke	1 small piece	4
215	Kung pao chicken	1 cup	16
216	Lamb stew	1 cup	5
217	Lamb, biryani	1 cup	12
218	Lemon grass chicken	1 cup	8
219	Liver pate	1 slice (4 1/4" x 1 1/2" x 1/2") or 2 oz.	3
220	Lo mein, with beef, chicken, or pork	1 cup	8
221	Moo goo gai pan	1 cup	7
222	Moo shoo pork	1/2 cup with 2 pancakes	10
223	Moussaka	1 piece (3" x 4")	12

#	Name	Amount	Points
224	Mushroom gravy and charbroiled beef patty, frozen	1 patty with gravy (5 3/4 oz.)	4
225	Noodles and sauce mix	1/2 cup prepared	3
226	Noodles, cellophane, cooked	1 cup	3
227	Noodles, egg	1 cup cooked or 1 1/2 oz. uncooked	3
228	Noodles, Oriental (bean thread)	1 cup prepared	4
229	Osso bucco	6 oz. veal with 1/4 cup sauce	13
230	Oyster stew, canned (made with low-fat or skim milk)	1 cup	3
231	Oyster stew, canned (made with whole milk)	1 cup	4
232	Pad Thai	1 cup	7
233	Paella	1 cup	7
234	Paprikash	2 cups (1 1/2 cups chicken mixture with 1/2 cup sauce)	9
235	Pastitsio	1 piece (3 1/4" x 3")	11

#	Name	Amount	Points
236	Peking duck	2 oz. duck with 1 piece duck skin and 3 pancakes	11
237	Pepper steak	6 oz.	13
238	Pico de gallo	1/2 cup	0
239	Pigs in blankets	2 (1 oz.)	6
240	Pimiento-cheese spread, reduced-fat, store-bought	2 tbsp. (1 oz.)	2
241	Pimiento-cheese spread, store-bought	2 tbsp. (1 oz.)	3
242	Pizza, crust dough, refrigerated, frozen, or ready-made	1 oz.	2
243	Pizza, Canadian-style bacon, frozen	1 slice (5 oz.)	7
244	Pizza, cheese, fast food, single serving	1	14
245	Pizza, cheese, frozen	1 slice (5 oz.)	8
246	Pizza, cheese, frozen, single serving	1 (7 oz.)	13

#	Name	Amount	Points
247	Pizza, cheese, thin or thick crust	1 slice (1/8 of 12" or 1/12 of 14"-16" pie)	4
248	Pizza, cheese, thin or thick crust	1 slice (1/8 of 18" pie)	9
249	Pizza, hamburger, pepperoni, sausage, or supreme, frozen	1 slice (5 oz.)	8
250	Pizza, pepperoni, sausage, or supreme, frozen, single serving	1 (7 oz.)	14
251	Pizza, pepperoni, thin or thick crust	1 slice (1/8 of 12" or 1/12 of 14"-16") pie)	5
252	Pizza, pepperoni, thin or thick crust	1 slice (1/8 of 18" pie)	10
253	Pizza, pieces, frozen (prepared without fat)	6 (3 oz.)	5
254	Pizza, vegetable, frozen	1 slice (5 oz.)	6
255	Pocket sandwich, frozen, any type	1 (4 1/2 oz.)	8
256	Poi	1/3 cup cooked (3 oz.)	1
257	Polenta	1/4 cup cooked (2 oz.)	4
258	Potato salad	1/2 cup	6

#	Name	Amount	Points
259	Potato salad, store-bought	1/2 cup (4 oz.)	4
260	Pozole (pork and hominy soup), canned	1 cup	3
261	Quenelles	8 (2 1/2" x 1 1/2" x 3/4") or 7 oz.	14
262	Quesadilla, beef	1 (1/2 of 6" diameter)	7
263	Quesadilla, cheese	1 (1/2 of 6" diameter)	5
264	Quesadilla, chicken	1 (1/2 of 6" diameter)	6
265	Quesadilla, vegetable	1 (1/2 of 6" diameter)	6
266	Quiche Lorraine	1/8 of 9" pie	12
267	Quiche Lorraine, frozen	1 serving (5 1/2 oz.)	10
268	Quiche, appetizer, frozen	2 (each 3/4 oz.)	3
269	Quiche, crab, frozen	1 serving (5 oz.)	11
270	Quiche, vegetable	1/8 of 9" pie	9
271	Quiche, vegetable, frozen	1 serving (5 oz.)	9
272	Ratatouille	1 cup	5
273	Ravioli, beef or chicken, without sauce, frozen	1 cup (4 oz.)	4
274	Ravioli, beef, breaded, frozen	6 (4 oz.)	5
275	Ravioli, beef, in meat sauce, canned	1 cup	5

#	Name	Amount	Points
276	Ravioli, cheese with tomato sauce	8 pieces or 1 cup with 1/2 cup sauce	16
277	Ravioli, cheese, breaded, frozen	6 (4 oz.)	7
278	Ravioli, cheese, without sauce, frozen	1 cup (4 oz.)	6
279	Ravioli, meat with tomato sauce	8 pieces or 1 cup with 1/2 cup tomato sauce	14
280	Ravioli, meat, without sauce	8 pieces or 1 cup with 1/2 cup tomato sauce	12
281	Reuben sandwich	1	17
282	Reuben sandwich	1	17
283	Rice noodles, packaged	1/2 cup prepared	3
284	Rice pilaf	1 cup	7
285	Risotto	1/2 cup	4
286	Saimin	1 cup	2
287	Salad dressing, fat-free (except Italian)	2 tbsp.	1
288	Salad dressing, fat-free, Italian	2 tbsp.	0
289	Salad dressing, reduced-calorie (except Italian)	2 tbsp.	2

69

#	Name	Amount	Points
290	Salad dressing, reduced-calorie, Italian	2 tbsp.	1
291	Salad dressing, regular, any type	2 tbsp.	4
292	Salad Nicoise, with dressing	4 cups	13
293	Salad Nicoise, without dressing	4 cups	5
294	Salad, grilled chicken, without dressing, fast food	1	4
295	Salad, mixed greens	1 cup	0
296	Salad, side, without dressing, fast food	1 serving	0
297	Satay	2 skewers with 1/4 cup sauce	9
298	Sauerbraten	3 oz. beef with 2 tbsp. gravy	6
299	Seitan	2 slices (2 oz.) or 2 tbsp. prepared mix	1
300	Sesame noodles	1 cup	7
301	Sesame sticks, store-bought	1/3 cup (1 oz.)	4

#	Name	Amount	Points
302	Shabu shabu	1 serving (4 oz. beef, 2 oz. tofu, and 1 1/2 cups vegetables)	8
303	Shish kabob	2 small skewers	10
304	Sloppy joe	1	8
305	Souffle, cheese	1 cup (6 oz.)	7
306	Souvalaki	1 large skewer	10
307	Souvalaki sandwich	1	7
308	Spaetzle	1/2 cup	4
309	Spinach, salad, with bacon, mushrooms, and dressing	2 cups	12
310	Spring roll, with beef, chicken, pork, or shrimp	1 (4 1/2" long)	4
311	Steak au poivre	6 oz. steak with 1 tbsp. sauce	15
312	Steak sandwich, frozen	1 (2 oz.)	5
313	Stuffing	1/2 cup	4
314	Stuffing mix, bread	1/2 cup prepared	4

#	Name	Amount	Points
315	Succotash	1 cup or 6 oz. cooked	2
316	Sukiyaki	2 1/2 cups	12
317	Sunomono	1/2 cup	1
318	Sushi, maki (vegetables and rice rolled in seaweed)	4 pieces	1
319	Sushi, nigiri (slicesd raw fish over rice>	4 pieces	3
320	Sushi, nori maki (raw fish and rice rolled in seaweed)	4 pieces	2
321	Swedish meatballs	6 (1" diameter)	8
322	Swedish meatballs with noodles, frozen	1 cup (6 1/2 oz.)	7
323	Tabouli	1/2 cup	4
324	Tabouli, from mix (prepared according to package directions)	1/2 cup prepared	2
325	Taco dinner kit in a box (prepared according to package directions)	2 tacos prepared	7

#	Name	Amount	Points
326	Taco salad shells, store-bought	2 small or 1 large (1 1/2 oz.)	5
327	Taco salad, with shell, without dressing, fast food	1	15
328	Taco salad, without shell and dressing, fast food	1	6
329	Taco shells, store-bought	2 (3/4 oz.)	2
330	Taco, beef or chicken	1	5
331	Taco, hard or soft, fast food	1	4
332	Tacos, soft, kit in a box (prepared according to package directions)	2	9
333	Tamale, beef, canned	2 (4 3/4 oz.)	5
334	Tamale, beef, frozen	3 small or 1 large (4 oz.)	7
335	Tamale, chicken, canned	2 (6 oz.)	3
336	Tamale, chicken, frozen	3 small or 1 large (4 1/2 oz.)	6
337	Tamale, pork, frozen	3 small or 1 large (4 1/2 oz.)	7

#	Name	Amount	Points
338	Tamales with sauce	2 (4" x 2")	10
339	Tandoori chicken, without skin	2 pieces (1 breast and 1 thigh)	8
340	Taquitos, frozen	2 (each 1 oz.)	3
341	Tempura batter mix	1/4 cup mix (1 oz.)	2
342	Tempura, shrimp	4 jumbo shrimp	11
343	Tempura, vegetable	1 cup	8
344	Teppan-yaki	1 1/2 cups	10
345	Teriyaki beef	2 slices (4 oz.)	7
346	Teriyaki chicken	2 slices (4 oz.)	6
347	Teriyaki fish	4 oz.	4
348	Thai crisp noodles	1 cup	11
349	Three bean salad, canned	1/2 cup (4 1/2 oz.)	1
350	Three-bean salad	1/2 cup	5
351	Tonkatsu	3/4 cup or 3 1/2 oz.	12
352	Tostada shells, store-bought	2 (3/4 oz.)	2
353	Tostada, filled, beef or chicken	1	8
354	Tuna salad	1/2 cup	6
355	Tuna salad sandwich	1	11
356	Tuna salad, store-bought	1/2 cup (3 1/2 oz.)	5

#	Name	Amount	Points
357	Turkey roll	1 slice (1 oz.)	1
358	Turkey tetrazzini	1 1/2 cups	9
359	Tzimmes, vegetables	3/4 cup	2
360	Veal marsala	4 oz.	11
361	Veal parmigiana, with sauce	5 oz. with 1/2 cup tomato sauce	12
362	Veal parmigiana, without sauce	1 serving (5 1/2 oz.)	10
363	Veal piccata	2 slices (4 oz.)	11
364	Veal scaloppine	2 pieces (each 3" x 5") or 4 1/2 oz.	12
365	Veal with peppers	5 oz.	11
366	Vegetarian breakfast links (sausage-type)	2 (1 1/2 oz.)	2
367	Vegetarian breakfast patty (sausage-type)	1 (1 oz.)	1
368	Vegetarian breakfast strips	4 (1 oz.)	3
369	Vegetarian burger	1 (2 3/4 oz.)	2
370	Vegetarian burger, black bean	1 (3 oz.)	2

#	Name	Amount	Points
371	Vegetarian burger, fat-free	1 (2 3/4 oz.)	1
372	Vegetarian burger, fat-free, high-fiber (5 grams or more dietary fiber per burger)	1 (2 3/4 oz.)	1
373	Vegetarian frankfurter, regular or fat-free	1 small or 1/2 large (1 1/2 oz.)	1
374	Vegetarian ground "meat", frozen	1/2 cup (2 oz.)	1
375	Vegetarian sausage, frozen	1 1/2 oz.	2
376	Vitello tonnato	2 slices veal (4 oz.) with 1/2 cup sauce	20
377	Waldorf salad	1/2 cup	6
378	Wiener schnitzel	4 oz.	11
379	Yakitori	1 skewer with 3 tbsp. sauce	6
380	Yam patty, frozen	1 (4 oz.)	1
381	Yams, sweetened, canned, in syrup	1 cup (9 oz.)	3
382	Yosenabe	2 cups	8
383	Ziti, baked	1 cup	5

Fats & Oils

#	Name	Amount	Points
1	Bacon fat	1 tbsp.	3
2	Brewer's yeast	1 tsp.	0
3	Creme fraiche	2 tbsp.	3
4	Lard	1 tbsp.	3
5	Oil, vegetable	1 tsp.	1
6	Oil, vegetable	1 cup	58
7	Textured vegetable protein	1/3 cup (3/4 oz. dry)	1
8	Vegetable oil	1 tsp.	1
9	Vegetable shortening	1 tsp.	1

Fish

#	Name	Amount	Points
1	Anchovies	6(3/4) or 1 tsp. paste	1
2	Bass, striped, coooked	1 fillet (6 oz.)	4
3	Bluefish, cooked	1 fillet (6 oz.)	4
4	Boullabaisse, any type	2 cups	7
5	Carp, cooked	1 fillet (6 oz.)	7
6	Catfish, cooked	1 fillet (6 oz.)	4
7	Cod, cooked	1 fillet (6 oz.)	4
8	Crayfish, canned	1/2 cup or 4 oz.	2
9	Crayfish, cooked	1/2 cup (2 oz.)	1
10	Fish amandine	1 fillett (6 oz.)	13
11	Fish, Anchovies, canned in oil, drained	6	1
12	Fish, Baked, stuffed	1 serving	8
13	Fish, Bass, striped, cooked	1 fillet (6 oz.)	5
14	Fish, Blackened	1 fillet (6 oz.)	12
15	Fish, Bluefish, cooked	1 fillet (6 oz.)	6
16	Fish, Carp, cooked	1 fillet (6 oz.)	7
17	Fish, Catfish, cooked	1 fillet (6 oz.)	6
18	Fish, Cod, cooked	1 fillet (6 oz.)	4
19	Fish, Dried	1 oz.	2

#	Name	Amount	Points
20	Fish, Eel	1 oz.	2
21	Fish, Flounder	1 fillet (6 oz.)	4
22	Fish, Fried	1 fillet (6 oz.)	12
23	Fish, Grouper	1 fillet (6 oz.)	4
24	Fish, Haddock, cooked	1 fillet (6 oz.)	4
25	Fish, Halibut, cooked	1 fillet (6 oz.)	5
26	Fish, Herring, cooked	1 oz.	1
27	Fish, Mackeral, canned	1/2 cup	3
28	Fish, Mackeral, cooked	1 fillet (6 oz.)	8
29	Fish, Mahimahi(dolphinfish), cooked	1 fillet (6 oz.)	4
30	Fish, Perch, cooked	6 oz.	4
31	Fish, Pike, cooked	1 fillet (6 oz.)	4
32	Fish, Pollock, cooked	6 oz.	4
33	Fish, Pompano, cooked	6 oz.	9
34	Fish, Rockfish, cooked	1 fillet (6 oz.)	4
35	Fish, Salmon, canned	1/2 cup (4 oz.)	4
36	Fish, Salmon, cooked	1 fillet (6 oz.)	7
37	Fish, Salmon, grilled, frozen	3 oz.	2
38	Fish, Salmon, smoked	1 oz.	1

#	Name	Amount	Points
39	Fish, Sardines, canned in oil, drained	5	3
40	Fish, Smelt, cooked	1 oz.	1
41	Fish, Snapper, cooked	1 fillet (6 oz.)	4
42	Fish, Sole, cooked	1 fillet (6 oz.)	4
43	Fish, Stuffed, frozen	1 (5 oz.)	5
44	Fish, Swordfish, cooked	1 steak (6 oz.)	4
45	Fish, Trout, cooked	1 fillet (6 oz.)	8
46	Fish, Trout, rainbow, cooked	1 fillet (6 oz.)	6
47	Fish, Tuna, canned in oil, drained	1/2 cup	5
48	Fish, Tuna, canned in water	1/2 cup	3
49	Fish, Tuna, cooked	1 fillet (6 oz.)	6
50	Fish, Tuna, grilled, frozen	1 oz.	2
51	Fish, Whitefish, smoked	2 oz.	1
52	Fish, Whiting, cooked	6 oz.	4
53	Grouper	1 fillet (6 oz.)	4
54	Haddock	1 fillet (6 oz.)	4
55	Halibut	1 fillet (6 oz.)	4
56	Herring fillets, store-bought	1/4 cup (2 oz.)	3

#	Name	Amount	Points
57	Herring, chopped	1/4 cup	4
58	Herring, cooked	1 oz.	2
59	Shark, cooked	1 steak (6 oz.)	4
60	Smelt, cooked	1 oz.	1
61	Sole, cooked	1 fillet (6 oz.)	4
62	Swordfish, cooked	1 steak (6 oz.)	4
63	Trout, rainbow, cooked	1 fillet (6 oz.)	4
64	Tuna dinner in a box (prepred according to package directions)	1 cup prepared	7
65	Tuna, canned in oil, drained	1/2 cup (4 oz.)	5
66	Tuna, canned in water, drained	1/2 cup (4 oz.)	3
67	Tuna, cooked	1 steak (6 oz.)	4
68	Tuna, grilled, frozen	3 oz.	2
69	Tuna-noodle casserole	1 cup	14
70	Whitefish and pike, large, store-bought	1(1 1/4 oz.)	2
71	Whitefish and pike, small, store-bought	2(1 oz.)	2
72	Whitefish salad, store-bought	1 1/2 oz.	5
73	Whiting, cooked	1 fillet (6 oz.)	4

Fruit

#	Name	Amount	Points
1	Apple,fresh	1 large (8 oz.)	2
2	Apple,fresh	1 small (4 oz.)	1
3	Apples, mountain	3 (2"x 1 7/8")	1
4	Apples,crab	2 oz. or 1/2 cup	1
5	Apricots,dried	6 halves (3/4 oz.)	1
6	Apricots,fresh	3 (4 oz.)	1
7	Apricots,unsweetened,canned	1 cup (9oz.)	2
8	Avacado	1/4 (2 oz.)	2
9	Avacado	1/4 (2 oz.)	2
10	Banana	1 medium (6 oz.)	2
11	Blackberries	1 cup (5 oz.)	1
12	Blueberries	1 cup (5 oz.)	1
13	Boysenberries	1 cup (5 oz.)	1
14	Breadfruit,uncooked	1 cup (8 oz.)	4
15	Cantaloupe	1/4 melon (8 oz.) or 1 cup (5 oz.)	1
16	Carambola (star fruit)	1 (5 oz.)	1
17	Casaba melon	1 cup (6 oz.)	1
18	Cherries,dried	1/4 cup (1 1/2 oz.)	2
19	Cherries,fresh	1 cup (5 1/2 oz.)	1

#	Name	Amount	Points
20	Coconut,cream of	1/4 cup (2 fl. oz.)	5
21	Coconut,shredded	1 tsp.	0
22	Currants,dried	1/4 cup (1 1/2 oz.)	2
23	Currants,fresh	1 cup (4 oz.)	1
24	Fig,dried	1 (3/4 oz.)	1
25	Fig,fresh	1 (2 oz.)	0
26	Fruit,candied	2 tbsp.	1
27	Fruit,dried,mixed	1/4 cup (1 1/2 oz.)	2
28	Fruit,spreadable	1 1/2 tbsp.	1
29	Gooseberries	1 cup (5 oz.)	1
30	Grapefruit	1 (16 oz.)	2
31	Grapefruit sections	1 cup (9 oz.)	1
32	Grapes	1 cup, 20 small or 12 large	1
33	Green papaya	1 cup	1
34	Guava	1 (4 oz.) or 1/3 pulp	1
35	Honeydew melon	1/8 (6 oz.) or 1 cup	1
36	Jackfruit	1/2 cup	2
37	Kiwi fruit	1 (4 oz.)	1

#	Name	Amount	Points
38	Kumquats	10 small or 5 medium (3 oz.)	1
39	Lichees,fresh	10 medium (6 oz.)	1
40	Loganberries	1 cup (5 oz.)	1
41	Loquats	10 (6 oz.)	1
42	Tangelo	1 (7 oz.)	1
43	Tangerine	1 (6 oz.)	1
44	Watermelon	2" slice or 1 cup (5 1/2 oz.)	1

Gelatins & Puddings

#	Name	Amount	Points
1	Banana Pudding	1 cup	7
2	Gelatin, fruit flavored	1/2 cup prepared	2
3	Gelatin, fruit flavored, sugar free	1/2 cup prepared	0
4	Gelatin-fruit mold	1/2 cup	3
5	Jam, jelly, or preserves	1 tbsp.	1
6	Jelly beans	10 (1 oz.)	2
7	Kugel, lukschen	1 piece (3" x 3 1/4")	7
8	Kugel, noodle, store-bought	1/2 cup (4 oz.)	3
9	Kugel, potato	1 piece (3" x 3 1/4")	3
10	Kugel, potato, store-bought	1/2 cup (3 1/2 oz.)	4
11	Pudding, any flavor	1 cup	7
12	Pudding, bread	1 cup	9
13	Pudding, Indian	1 cup	12
14	Pudding, plum	1/2 cup with 1 tbsp. sauce	12
15	Pudding, ready-made	1/2 cup	4
16	Pudding, ready-made, reduced-calorie	1/2 cup	2
17	Pudding, reduced-calorie (made with skim, nonfat, or low-fat [1%] milk)	1 cup	2
18	Pudding, rice	1 cup	7
19	Pudding, tapioca	1 cup	6

Grains & Rices

#	Name	Amount	Points
1	Barley	1 cup cooked or 1/4 cup uncooked	3
2	Bran, Corn, uncooked	1/4 cup	0
3	Bran, Oat, uncooked	1/4 cup	1
4	Bran, Rice, uncooked	1/4 cup	2
5	Bran, Wheat, uncooked	1 tbsp.	0
6	Bran, Wheat, uncooked	1/4 cup	0
7	Bulgur, uncooked	1/4 cup	2
8	Corn dog	1 (2 3/4 oz.)	5
9	Corn on the cob	1 small ear (5") or 4 oz.	1
10	Corn, baby (ears)	1 cup	1
11	Corn, kernels or cream-style	1 cup (6 oz.)	2
12	Cornstarch	1 tsp.	1
13	Flour, any type	1 tsp.	0
14	Flour, any type	3 tbsp. (3/4 oz.)	1
15	Flour, Potato	1 tsp.	0
16	Flour, Potato	1/4 cup	2
17	Flour, White	1 cup	9
18	Flour, White	3 tbsp.	1
19	Flour, White	1 tsp.	0

#	Name	Amount	Points
20	Flour, Whole Wheat	1 cup	8
21	Flour, Whole Wheat	3 tbsp.	1
22	Flour, Whole Wheat	1 tsp.	0
23	Rice (crisp) and marshmallow treat	1 small (3/4 oz.)	2
24	Rice dirty	1 cup	9
25	Rice mix, flavored, any type	1/2 cup prepared	3
26	Rice, dirty, mix (prepared without fat)	1 cup prepared	3
27	Rice, fried, chicken or pork, frozen	1 cup	2
28	Rice, fried, with beef, chicken, pork, or shrimp	1/2 cup	8
29	Rice, Spanish	1 cup	5
30	Rice, Spanish, canned	1 cup (9 oz.)	3
31	Rice, white	1 cup	4
32	Rice, wild	1 cup cooked	3
33	Seeds, caraway	1 tsp.	0
34	Seeds, poppy	1 tsp.	0
35	Seeds, pumpkin or sunflower	1 tbsp.	1
36	Seeds, sesame	1 tsp.	0

Herbs & Spices

#	Name	Amount	Points
1	Caraway seeds	1 tsp.	0
2	Caraway seeds	1 tbsp.	0
3	Chili with beans, canned	1 cup (9 oz.)	8
4	Chili without beans, canned	1 cup (8 1/2 oz.)	11
5	Chili, bean, in a cup	1 (2 oz. dry)	3
6	Chili, frozen	1 cup (8 oz.)	12
7	Chili, low-fat, canned	1 cup (9 oz.)	4
8	Chili, turkey, with beans, canned	1 cup (8 1/2 oz.)	3
9	Chili, turkey, without beans, canned	1 cup (8 1/2 oz.)	3
10	Chili, vegetarian, low-fat or fat-free (5 grams or more dietary fiber per cup)	1 cup	2
11	Chili, vegetarian, low-fat or fat-free, canned	1 cup	3
12	Elderberries	1 cup (5 oz.)	1
13	Fennel (anise, sweet anise, or finocchio)	1 cup or 1 oz.	0
14	Gobo (burdock)	1/2 cup (2 oz.)	1
15	Grape leaves	1 cup	0

#	Name	Amount	Points
16	Horseradish tree leaves (marongay)	1 cup or 1 oz.	0
17	Horseradish, prepared	1 tbsp.	0
18	Jalapenos, stuffed (prepared without fat)	2 (each 1 oz.)	4
19	Pepper, bell	1 cup, 1 medium or 4 oz.	0
20	Pepper, chili	1 cup, 1 medium or 6 oz.	0
21	Pepper, jalapeno, canned	1 cup or 6 oz.	0
22	Pepper, stuffed with beef and rice	1	6
23	Pepper, stuffed with beef, in tomato sauce, frozen	1 with sauce (7 oz.)	4
24	Prickly pear (cactus pear)	1 (5 oz.)	1

Meats

#	Name	Amount	Points
1	Antelope, cooked	1 oz.	1
2	Armadillo, cooked	1 oz.	1
3	Bacon, Canadian-style	1 slice (1 oz.)	1
4	Bacon, cooked, crisp	3 slices	3
5	Bacon, reduced-fat, cooked, crisp	3 slices	3
6	Bacon, turkey, cooked, crisp	3 slices	2
7	Bear, black, cooked	1 oz.	2
8	Beaver, cooked	1 oz.	1
9	Beef and Broccoli	1 cup	4
10	Beef and broccoli, frozen	1 cup (7 oz.)	5
11	Beef Bourguignon	1 1/2 cups	18
12	Beef jerky or stick	1 oz.	3
13	Beef, Bourguignon	1 1/2 cups	20
14	Beef, corned, canned	1 slice (2 oz.)	3
15	Beef, dried, store-bought	7 slices (1 oz.)	1
16	Beef, Ground, country-fried, store-bought	1 patty(4 oz.)	8
17	Beef, Ground, lean, cooked	1 patty (3 oz.)	6
18	Beef, Ground, lean, cooked	1/2 cup (2 oz.)	4

#	Name	Amount	Points
19	Beef, Ground, lean, cooked(round or loin cuts with all visible fat trimmed)	1 slice or 1/2 cup cubed or shredded (2 oz.)	3
20	Beef, Ground, lean, uncooked	1 pound	22
21	Beef, Ground, regular, cooked	1 patty (3 oz.)	6
22	Beef, Ground, regular, cooked	1/2 cup (2 oz.)	4
23	Beef, Ground, regular, cooked	1 patty (3 oz.)	6
24	Beef, Ground, regular, uncooked	1 pound	25
25	Beef, Orange-Ginger	1 cup	11
26	Beef, regular, cooked	1 slice or 1/2 cup cubed or shredded (2 oz.)	4
27	Beef, steak, cooked	1 small (4 oz.)	7
28	Beef, steak, cooked	1 small (4 oz.)	7
29	Beef, steak, lean (round or loin cuts with all visible fat trimmed), cooked	1 small (4 oz.)	5
30	Beef, steak, lean (round or loin cuts with all visible fat trimmed), cooked	1 small (4 oz.)	5

#	Name	Amount	Points
31	Beef, Sweet and sour	1 cup	12
32	Beef, Tongue, cooked	1 oz.	2
33	Beefalo, cooked	1 oz.	1
34	Bologna, beef or pork	1 slice (1 oz.)	2
35	Bologna, turkey	1 slice (1 oz.)	1
36	Boudin, store-bought	2 oz.	2
37	Bratwurst	2 oz.	5
38	Buffalo, water cooked	1 oz.	1
39	Caribou, cooked	1 oz.	1
40	Chitterlings	1 oz.	2
41	Chorizo	1 link (5" long) or 3 1/2 oz.	9
42	Crab, deviled	1/2 cup	5
43	Crab, stuffed, frozen	1 (3 oz.)	3
44	Crabmeat, artificial	1/2 cup (3 oz.)	2
45	Crabmeat, canned	1/2 cup or 4 oz.	2
46	Crabmeat, cooked	1/2 cup (2 oz.)	1
47	Duck a l orange	1/4 duck with 2 tsbp. sauce	19
48	Duck with fruit sauce	1/4 duck with skin and 1/2 cup sauce	13

#	Name	Amount	Points
49	Duck, wild or domestic, with skin, cooked	1/4 duck (3 1/2 oz. without bone)	13
50	Duck, wild or domestic, without skin, cooked	1/4 duck (3 1/2 oz. without bone)	5
51	Elk, cooked	1 oz.	1
52	Emu, cooked	1 oz.	1
53	Flanken	2 slices (4 oz.)	8
54	Frankfurter, beef and pork, with cheese	1 (1 3/4 oz.)	5
55	Frankfurter, beef and pork, fat-free	1 (1 3/4 oz.)	1
56	Frankfurter, beef and pork, light	1 (1 3/4 oz.)	2
57	Frankfurter, beef and pork, regular	1 (1 3/4 oz.)	5
58	Frankfurter, chicken	1 (2 oz.)	4
59	Frankfurter, Rolls, light	1 (1 1/2 oz.)	2
60	Frankfurter, Rolls, reduced-calorie	1 (1 1/2 oz.)	1
61	Frankfurter, Rolls, regular	1 (1 1/2 oz.)	3
62	Frankfurter, turkey	1 (2 oz.)	3
63	Frankfurter, turkey, fat-free	1 (1 1/2 oz.)	1

#	Name	Amount	Points
64	Frankfurter, turkey, light	1 (2 oz.)	3
65	Frog's legs, fried	2 (3 oz. with bone)	4
66	Gizzards, cooked	1 oz.	1
67	Goat meat, cooked	1 oz.	1
68	Goose, wild, cooked	1 oz.	1
69	Guinea hen, cooked	1 oz.	1
70	Ham, cooked	1 slice, 1/2 cup cubed or shredded or 2 oz.	3
71	Hash, corned beef, canned	1 cup	10
72	Hash, roast beef, canned	1 cup	9
73	Heart, Beef, cooked	1 oz.	1
74	Hunan Beef	1 cup	9
75	Kidney, cooked	1/2 cup (2 oz.)	2
76	Knockwurst	2 oz.	5
77	Lamb, ground, cooked	1/2 cup (2 oz.)	4
78	Lamb, lean (leg and loin cuts with all visible fat trimmed), cooked	1 slice, 1chop, 1/2 cup cubed or shredded or 2 oz.	3
79	Lamb, regular, cooked	1 slice, 1 chop, 1/2 cup cubed or shredded or 2 oz.	4

#	Name	Amount	Points
80	Liver with bacon	2 slices (4 oz.)	9
81	Liver with onions	2 slices (4 oz.)	7
82	Liver, beef, cooked	1 slice or 1/2 cup (2 oz.)	2
83	Liver, chopped	1/4 cup	5
84	Liverwurst	1 oz.	3
85	Luncheon meat, canned	2 oz.	5
86	Luncheon meat, canned, light	2 oz.	3
87	Luncheon meat, fat-free	2 oz.	1
88	Luncheon meat, lean (less than 2g fat per oz), 1 slice or 1 oz.	1 slice or 1 oz.	1
89	Luncheon meat, regular(4 grams fat or more per oz.)	1 slice (1 oz.)	2
90	Vienna sausage, chicken, canned	3 (1/2 oz.)	3
91	Vietnamese beef balls(Thit bo vien)	6 (1 1/2 oz.)	2

Nuts, Seeds & Butters

#	Name	Amount	Points
1	Almond butter	1 tsp.	1
2	Almonds	22 nuts (1 oz. shelled)	4
3	Brazil nuts	8 nuts (1 oz. shelled)	5
4	Butter,regular	1 cup	51
5	Butter,regular or whipped	1 tsp.	1
6	Cashews,dry-roasted,without salt added	14 nuts (1 oz. shelled)	4
7	Chestnuts	6 small (2 oz.)	1
8	Dates,dried	1/4 cup (5 dates)	2
9	Dates,fresh	2 (3/4 oz.)	1
10	Fruit butter,any type	1 tbsp.	1
11	Hazelnuts	20 nuts (1 oz. shelled)	4
12	Pistachios	40 nuts (1 oz. shelled)	4
13	Soybean nuts	1/4 cup (1 oz.)	3
14	Walnuts	14 halves (1 oz. shelled)	5

Pasta

#	Name	Amount	Points
1	Cannelloni, cheese, with meat sauce	2 shells with 1/2 cup sauce	29
2	Cannelloni, cheese, with tomato sauce	2 shells with 1/2 cup a of sauce	14
3	Cannelloni, meat, with cream sauce	2 shells with 1/2 cup sauce	17
4	Cannelloni, meat, with tomato sauce	2 shells with 1/2 cup sauce	14
5	Cannelloni, spinach and cheese, with cream sauce	2 shells with 1/2 cup sauce	15
6	Cannelloni, spinach and cheese, with tomato sauce	2 shells with 1/2 cup sauce	12
7	Cannelloni, with tomato sauce, frozen	7 oz.	6
8	Fettuccini Alfredo	1 cup	16
9	Fettuccini Alfredo, frozen	1 cup (7 oz.)	7
10	Fettuccini with broccoli and chicken in Alfredo sauce, frozen	1 cup (8 oz.)	9
11	Lasagna, cheese, with tomato sauce, frozen	1 package (10 oz.)	8

#	Name	Amount	Points
12	Lasagna, chicken, frozen	1 cup (7 oz.)	5
13	Lasagna, vegetable, frozen	1 cup (7 1/2 oz.)	5
14	Lasagna, vegetable, frozen	1 cup	5
15	Lasagna, vegetarian, with cheese	1 serving	10
16	Lasagna, vegetarian, with cheese and spinach	1 serving	9
17	Lasagna, with meat	1 cup	6
18	Lasagna, with meat sauce, frozen	1 cup (7 1/2 oz.)	6
19	Lasgana noodles, uncooked	2 1/2 or 2 oz.	4
20	Linguine, with red clam sauce	1 cup linguine with 1/2 cup sauce	6
21	Linguine, with white clam sauce	1 cup linguine with 1/2 cup sauce	8
22	Spaghetti with tomato sauce and meatballs	1 cup spaghetti with 1/2 cup sauce	12
23	Tortellini, beef, chicken, or pork, without sauce, frozen	1 cup (3 3/4 oz.)	5
24	Tortellini, cheese, without sauce	10 (2/3 cup)	3
25	Tortellini, cheese, without sauce, frozen	1 cup (3 3/4 oz.)	6
26	Tortellini, meat, without sauce	10 (2/3 cup)	3
27	Tortellini, mushroom, without sauce, frozen	1 cup (3 1/2 oz.)	6
28	Tortellini, sausage, without sauce, frozen	1 cup (3 3/4 oz.)	7

Poultry

#	Name	Amount	Points
1	Chicken thigh, fried, with skin (with bone)	1 (3 oz.)	6
2	Chicken thigh, fried, with skin, fast food	1	8
3	Chicken wing, fried, with skin, fast food	1	5
4	Cornish hen, with skin, cooked	1/2 hen	9
5	Cornish hen, without skin, cooked	1/2 hen	4
6	Heart, Chicken, cooked	1 oz.	1
7	Livers, chicken, cooked	1/2 cup (2 oz.)	2

Seafood

#	Name	Amount	Points
1	Abalone, cooked	3 oz.	2
2	Caviar or any type fish roe	2 tbsp. (1 oz.)	2
3	Clams, baked	6	8
4	Clams, canned	1/2 cup or 4 oz.	2

#	Name	Amount	Points
5	Clams, cooked	1/2 cup (2 oz.)	1
6	Clams, fried	1 cup	15
7	Clams, fried, frozen (prepared without fat)	3 oz.	6
8	Clams, stuffed, frozen (prepared without fat)	1 (3 oz.)	3
9	Coquilles St. Jacques	2 shells	9
10	Gumbo, seafood, with rice	1 cup	3
11	Gumbo, seafood, with rice, store-bought	1 cup (9 oz.)	5
12	Gumbo, with rice mix	1/4 cup mix (1 1/2 oz.)	3
13	Lo mein, with shrimp	1 cup	8
14	Lobster Cantonese	1 cup	9
15	Lobster meat, canned	1/2 cup or 4 oz.	2
16	Lobster meat, cooked	1/2 cup (2 oz.)	1
17	Lobster Newburg	1 cup	11
18	Lobster salad	1/2 cup	4
19	Lobster salad sandwich	1	8

#	Name	Amount	Points
20	Lobster thermidor	1 cup	16
21	Lobster, roll sandwich	1	5
22	Lobster, steamed	1 (1 1/4 pound lobster or 4 1/2 oz. lobster meat)	3
23	Shrimp scampi	9 medium shrimp (3 oz.)	11
24	Shrimp toast	1 piece	2
25	Squid, cooked	3 oz.	2

Snacks

#	Name	Amount	Points
1	Bagel chips	1 oz.	3
2	Bagel chips,fat-free	1 oz.	2
3	Banana chips	1 oz.	3
4	Biscotti	8 mini,2 small or 1 regular (1 oz.)	3
5	Biscotti,chocolate	8 mini,2 small or 1 regular (1 oz.)	3
6	Biscotti,fat-free	8 mini,2 small or 1 regular (1 oz.)	2
7	Biscuit with sausage,fast-food	1	12
8	Biscuit,cheese	1	5
9	Biscuit,homemade	1 small (2" diameter)	3
10	Biscuit,refrigerated,baked	1 small (2 1/2" diameter) or 1/2 large	2
11	Corn nuts	1/2 cup (1 1/2 oz.)	4
12	Cornmeal mix,self-rising	2 tbsp. (3/4 oz.)	1
13	Cornmeat,cooked	1/4 cup (2 oz.)	4
14	Cornmeat,uncooked	2 tbsp. (1/2 oz.)	1
15	Crab puffs	6 (1 1/2" rounds)	7

#	Name	Amount	Points
16	Crab Rangoon	1 large (4 1/2") or 5 mini	4
17	Crab Rangoon,frozen	8 (5 1/4 oz.)	11
18	Crackers,snack,with filling (cheese,wheat,rye,toast, or wafer crackers with cheese,peanut butter, or cream cheese filling)	6 (1 1/4 oz.)	5
19	Croquettes,beef	2 (each 2 1/2 oz.)	10
20	Croquettes,chicken	2 (each 2 1/2 oz.)	9
21	Croutons,homemade	1/2 cup	4
22	Croutons,packaged	1/2 cup (1 oz.)	3
23	Croutons,packaged,fat-free	1/2 cup (1 oz.)	2
24	Egg roll snacks,pork,shrimp, or vegetable,store-bought	3 oz.	3
25	French fries	20 (each about 4 1/2" long) or 2 oz.)	10
26	French fries,fast food	1 large serving	13
27	French fries,fast food	1 medium serving	10
28	French fries,fast food	1 small serving	6

#	Name	Amount	Points
29	French fries,frozen,baked	15 (3 oz.)	2
30	French toast	2 slices	7
31	French toast sticks,fast food,without syrup	6	12
32	French toast sticks,frozen	3 (2 1/2 oz.)	6
33	French toast,frozen,baked	2 slices (4 oz.)	5
34	Fritters,corn	3 (each 2 1/2" x 2")	5
35	Fritters,vegetable	1 cup	10
36	Granola bar,any type other than chocolate-covered	1 (1 oz.)	3
37	Granola bar,chocolate-covered	1 (1 1/3 oz.)	4
38	Granola bar,reduced-calorie	1 (1 oz.)	2
39	Gum,chewing,with sugar or sugarless	1 stick or piece	0
40	Ham and cheese sandwich,grilled	1	15
41	Hamantaschen	1 piece (3" diameter)	3
42	Hamburger,Large,fast-food	1	13
43	Hamburger,microwave,frozen	1 small (1 1/2 oz.)	3
44	Hamburger,microwave,frozen	1 small (1 1/2 oz.)	3

#	Name	Amount	Points
45	Hamburger,Small,fast-food	1	6
46	Hamburger,without mayonnaise,lettuce & tomato	1	9
47	Ice pop,fruit-flavored	1 (1 3/4 fl. oz.)	1
48	Italian toast snacks,store-bought	4 (1 oz.)	3
49	Knish,any type	1 (3 1/2" square)	6
50	Knish,potato,store-bought	1 (4 1/2 oz.)	3
51	Kreplachs,boiled	2 (each 4" x 3" x 3")	5
52	Kreplachs,fried	2 (each 4" x 3" x 3")	7
53	Kreplachs,frozen	4 (3 oz.)	4
54	Licorice	1 oz.	2
55	Lollipop	1 (2 1/4" diameter)	1
56	Melba toast,all varieties	6 rounds or 4 slices (3/4 oz.)	1

Soups, Sauces & Gravies

#	Name	Amount	Points
1	Adobo sauce, light, store-bought	1/2 cup	5
2	Adobo sauce, store-bought	1 Tbsp (1/2 oz.)	2
3	Alfredo sauce, light, store-bought	1/2 cup (4 oz.)	5
4	Alfredo sauce, store-bought	1/2 cup (4 oz.)	10
5	Applesauce, unsweetened	1 cup (8 oz.)	1
6	Avgolemono soup	1 cup	3
7	Barbeque sauce	1 tbsp.	0
8	Barbeque sauce	1/4 cup	1
9	Bean and bacon soup, canned	1 cup	3
10	Bean and ham soup, canned	1 cup	3
11	Bearnaise sauce	1/4 cup	8
12	Bearnaise sauce, store-bought	1/4 cup (2 oz.)	10
13	Bechamel (white) sauce	1/4 cup	4
14	Beef broth and tomato juice	1 cup (8 fl. oz.)	2
15	Beef in barbeque sauce, frozen	1/4 cup (2 oz.)	3

#	Name	Amount	Points
16	Beef noodle soup mix, single serving	1 cup prepared	4
17	Beef soup, canned	1 cup	2
18	Beef vegetable soup, canned	1 cup	1
19	Black bean sauce	1 tsp.	0
20	Black bean soup	1 cup	4
21	Black bean soup in a cup	1 (2 oz. dry)	3
22	Black bean soup, canned	1 cup	2
23	Bolognese meat sauce	1/2 cup	6
24	Borscht, Beet,	1 cup with 2 tbsp. sour cream	4
25	Borscht, low-calorie, store-bought	1 cups	0
26	Borscht, store-bought	1 cup	2
27	Boullion, any type	1 cup	0

#	Name	Amount	Points
28	Broccoli soup, cream of, canned(made with whole milk)	1 cup	4
29	Broccoli soup, cream of	1 cup	5
30	Broccoli soup, cream of, canned(made with low-fat or skim milk)	1 cup	3
31	Broccoli soup, cream of, low-fat, canned(made with low-fat or skim milk)	1 cup	3
32	Broccoli, cheese soup, canned (made with low-fat or skim milk)	1 cup	3
33	Broccoli, cheese soup, canned (made with whole milk)	1 cup	4
34	Broccoli, cheese soup, low-fat, canned(made with low-fat or skim milk)	1 cup	2
35	Broth, any type	1 cup	0
36	Cabbage soup	1 cup	2

#	Name	Amount	Points
37	Celery soup, cream of, low-fat, canned(made with low-fat or skim milk)	1 cup	2
38	Celery soup, cream of, canned(made with low-fat or skim milk)	1 cup	3
39	Celery soup, cream of, canned(made with whole milk)	1 cup	4
40	Cheese sauce	1/4 cup	2
41	Cheese sauce, store-bought	1/4 cup (2 1/4 oz.)	5
42	Chicken and stars soup, canned	1 cup	1
43	Chicken noodle soup	1 cup	3
44	Chicken noodle soup in a cup	1 (1 oz. dry)	2
45	Chicken noodle soup mix	1 cup prepared	2
46	Chicken noodle soup mix, single serving	1 cup prepared	4
47	Chicken noodle soup, canned	1 cup	2
48	Chicken soup, cream of, canned (made with low-fat or skim milk)	1 cup	4

#	Name	Amount	Points
49	Chicken soup, cream of, canned (made with whole milk)	1 cup	5
50	Chicken soup, cream of, low-fat, canned (made with low-fat or skim milk)	1 cup	3
51	Chicken soup, hot and spicy	1 cup	4
52	Chicken soup, with matzo balls	1 cup soup with 2 (1 1/2") matzo balls	3
53	Chicken soup, without matzo balls	1 cup	1
54	Chicken vegetable soup in a cup	1 (1 oz. dry)	2
55	Chicken with rice soup, canned	1 cup	2
56	Chicken with wild rice soup, canned	1 cup	2
57	Chili sauce, bottled	1 tbsp	0
58	Chili sauce, green or red	1/4 cup	1
59	Clam sauce, red	1/2 cup	3
60	Clam sauce, red, store-bought	1/2 cup (4 1/2 oz.)	2
61	Clam sauce, white	1/2 cup	9
62	Clam sauce, white, store-bought	1/2 cup (4 1/4 oz.)	3

#	Name	Amount	Points
63	Coconut ginger soup, Thai, canned	1 cup	3
64	Corn chowder soup in a cup	1 (1 oz. dry)	3
65	Corn chowder, canned (made with low-fat or skim milk)	1 cup	4
66	Corn chowder, canned (made with whole milk)	1 cup	5
67	Cranberry sauce	1/4 cup	2
68	Curry, beef, chicken, or lamb	1 cup	9
69	Donair sauce	2 tbsp.	2
70	Duck sauce	1 tbsp.	1
71	Egg drop soup	1 cup	1
72	Enchilada sauce	1/2 cup (4 oz.)	1
73	Escarole soup, canned	1 cup	1
74	Fondue, cheese	1/2 cup fondue with 2 oz. bread	12
75	Gazpacho	1 cup	5
76	Gazpacho, canned	1 cup	1
77	Gravy and salisbury steak, frozen	1 steak with gravy (4 3/4 oz.)	4

#	Name	Amount	Points
78	Gravy and sliced beef, canned	1/2 cup (5 oz.)	6
79	Gravy and sliced beef, frozen	2 slices with gravy (4 3/4 oz.)	2
80	Gravy and sliced turkey, frozen	2 slices with gravy (4 3/4 oz.)	2
81	Gravy, beef, chicken or turkey, canned	1/4 cup	1
82	Gravy, brown	1/4 cup	2
83	Gravy, cream	1/4 cup	3
84	Gravy, fat-free, canned	1/2 cup	1
85	Gravy, sausage, canned	1/4 cup	2
86	Hoisin sauce	1 tsp.	0
87	Hollandaise sauce	1/4 cup	8
88	Hollandaise sauce, store-bought	1/4 cup (2 oz.)	4
89	Horseradish sauce, store-bought	2 tbsp. (1 oz.)	3
90	Hot and sour soup	1 cup	2
91	Hot dog sauce	1/4 cup (2 oz.)	1
92	Kung pao sauce	2 tbsp.	1
93	Lentil soup	1 cup	3
94	Lentil soup in a cup	1 (2 oz. dry)	3
95	Lentil soup, canned	1 cup	2

#	Name	Amount	Points
96	Lobster bisque	1 cup	5
97	Lobster bisque, canned, made with low-fat or skim milk	1 cup	2
98	Lobster bisque, canned, made with whole milk	1 cup	3
99	Manhattan clam chowder	1 cup	5
100	Manhattan clam chowder, canned	1 cup	2
101	Manicotti shells, dry	2 (1 oz.)	2
102	Manicotti with meat sauce	2 shells with 1/2 cup sauce	15
103	Manicotti with tomato sauce	2 shells with 1/2 cup sauce	11
104	Manicotti, cheese, without sauce, frozen	2 (5 1/2 oz.)	6
105	Manicotti, cheese, wtih tomato sauce, frozen	1 package (10 oz.)	8
106	Marinara sauce	1/2 cup	3
107	Marinara sauce, store-bought	1/2 cup (4 1/2 oz.)	2
108	Minestrone soup	1 cup	4
109	Minestrone soup in a cup	1 (1 1/2 oz. dry)	2

#	Name	Amount	Points
110	Minestrone soup, canned	1 cup	2
111	Minestrone soup, low-fat, canned	1 cup	2
112	Miso soup	1 cup	2
113	Mole sauce, brown, store-bought	2 tbsp. (1 oz.)	4
114	Mole sauce, green, store-bought	2 tbsp. (1 oz.)	4
115	Mornay sauce	1/4 cup	4
116	Muligatawny soup	1 cup	5
117	Mushroom soup, cream of	1 cup	8
118	Mushroom soup, cream of, canned (made with low-fat or skim milk)	1 cup	3
119	Mushroom soup, cream of, canned (made with whole milk)	1 cup	4
120	Mushroom soup, cream of, low-fat, canned (made with low-fat or skim milk)	1 cup	2
121	Mushroom-barley soup	1 cup	5
122	Nam Prik	1 tbsp.	1
123	Nebeyaki udon	2 cups	8

#	Name	Amount	Points
124	New England clam chowder	1 cup	5
125	New England clam chowder, canned (made with low-fat or skim milk)	1 cup	3
126	New England clam chowder, canned (made with whole milk)	1 cup	4
127	New England clam chowder, low-fat, canned (made with low-fat or skim milk)	1 cup	2
128	Nuoc cham	1 tbsp.	0
129	Onion soup mix	1 cup prepared or 1/2 envelope	1
130	Onion soup, French, au gratin	1 cup	6
131	Oriental soup in a cup	1 (1 oz. dry)	2
132	Oriental soup mix, single-serving	1 cup prepared	7
133	Oyster sauce	1 tsp.	0
134	Pasta soup with vegetables, canned	1 cup	2
135	Peanut sauce, Thai, canned	2 tbsp. (1 oz.)	1
136	Pepperoni	1 oz.	4

#	Name	Amount	Points
137	Persian noodle soup, store-bought	1 cup	3
138	Persian pomegranate soup, store-bought	1 cup	4
139	Pesto sauce	2 tbsp.	3
140	Pesto sauce, store-bought	2 tbsp. (1 oz.)	3
141	Petite marmite	2 cup	7
142	Pizza sauce	1/4 cup (2 oz.)	1
143	Plum sauce	2 tbsp.	2
144	Potato soup, cream of	1 cup	2
145	Potato soup, cream of, canned (made with low-fat or skim milk)	1 cup	3
146	Potato soup, cream of, canned (made with whole milk)	1 cup	4
147	Potato soup, frozen	1 package (7 1/2 oz.)	2
148	Potato starch or flour	3 tbsp.	2
149	Potato starch or flour	1 tsp.	0
150	Ramen noodle soup mix	3 oz. dry	8
151	Ramen noodle soup mix, low-fat	3 oz. package prepared	6
152	Ramen soup in a cup, low-fat	1 (2 oz. dry)	3
153	Red beans and rice soup in a cup	1 (2 oz. dry)	3

#	Name	Amount	Points
154	Remoulade sauce	1 tbsp.	2
155	Roux, store-bought	1 tbsp.	5
156	Salsa	1/2 cup	0
157	Salsa con queso	2 tbsp. (1 oz.)	2
158	Schav, canned	1 cup	0
159	Sloppy joe sauce, store-bought	1/4 cup (2 oz.)	1
160	Soup, high-fiber, canned (7 grams or more dietary fiber per cup)	1 cup	1
161	Soy sauce	1 tbsp.	0
162	Spaghetti sauce, botted, any type, reduced-fat	1/2 cup (4 1/2 oz.)	1
163	Spaghetti sauce, bottled, any type	1/2 cup (4 1/2 oz.)	2
164	Spanish sauce	1/2 cup	1
165	Split pea soup	1 cup	4
166	Split pea soup in a cup	1 (2 oz. dry)	3
167	Split pea soup, canned	1 cup	3
168	Split pea soup, frozen	1 cup	2
169	Steak sauce	1 tbsp.	0
170	Suimono	1 cup	1
171	Sweet and sour sauce	2 tbsp.	1
172	Taco sauce	1 tbsp.	0

#	Name	Amount	Points
173	Tamari sauce	1 tbsp.	0
174	Tartar sauce	1 tbsp.	2
175	Tartar sauce, fat-free	1/4 cup	1
176	Teriyaki sauce	1 tbsp.	0
177	Teriyaki sauce	1/4 cup	1
178	Tom yum kung	1 cup	2
179	Tomato paste, canned	1/4 cup (2 oz.)	0
180	Tomato puree, canned	1/2 cup (4 oz.)	0
181	Tomato sauce, canned	1/2 cup	0
182	Tomato sauce, Italian	1/2 cup	2
183	Tomato shells (no pulp)	2	0
184	Tomato soup	1 cup	2
185	Tomato soup, canned (made with low-fat or skim milk)	1 cup	2
186	Tomato soup, canned (made with water)	1 cup	1
187	Tomato soup, canned (made with whole milk)	1 cup	3
188	Tomato soup, cream of	1 cup	5

#	Name	Amount	Points
189	Turkey noodle soup, canned	1 cup	1
190	Vegetable barley soup, frozen	1 package (7 1/2 oz.)	1
191	Vegetable beef soup, canned	1 cup	1
192	Vegetable soup	1 cup	3
193	Vegetable soup mix	1 cup prepared	1
194	Vegetable soup, canned	1 cup	2
195	Vegetarian vegetable soup in a cup	1 (1 1/2 oz. dry)	3
196	Vichyssoise	1 cup	5
197	Vindaloo, chicken	1 cup	8
198	Vindaloo, pork	1 cup	9
199	Wine sauce	1/4 cup	3
200	Wonton soup	1 cup with 4 wontons	4
201	Zuppa di pesce	2 cups	12

Soy Foods

#	Name	Amount	Points
1	Flour, soy	1/4 cup	2
2	Soy flour	3 tbsp.	2
3	Soy yogurt, flavored	3/4 cup (6 oz.)	3
4	Soy yogurt, plain	3/4 cup (6 oz.)	3
5	Tempeh (fermented soybean cake)	1/4 cup (1 oz.)	1
6	Tofu, any type	1/3 cup	2
7	Tofu, frozen	1/2 cup	5
8	Tofu, low-fat	1/3 cup	1

Vegetables

#	Name	Amount	Points
1	Arugula	1 cup	0
2	Asparagus, cooked	1 cup (6 oz.) or 12 spears	0
3	Bamboo shoots	1 cup	0
4	Beets, cooked	1 cup ((6 oz.)	0

#	Name	Amount	Points
5	Bittermelon (balsam-pear pods)	1 cup, cooked	0
6	Bittermelon (balsam-pear pods)	1 cup, uncooked	0
7	Bottle gourd	1 cup	0
8	Broccoli rabe	1 cup	0
9	Broccoli, cooked or uncooked	1 cup or 4 spears	0
10	Brussel sprouts, cooked or uncooked	1 cup (5 oz.)	0
11	Cabbage(all varieties including bok choy, kai choi, won bok, makina, Chinese, swamp, and mustard), cooked or uncooked	1 cup	0
12	Capers	1 tbsp.	0
13	Cardoon	1 cup	0
14	Carob, unsweetened	1 tsp.	0
15	Carrot and raisin salad	1/2 cup	5
16	Carrots and parsnips	1 cup	4
17	Carrots, cooked or uncooked	1 cup	1
18	Cauliflower, cooked or uncooked	1 cup (4 oz.)	0
19	Celeriac (celery root)	1 cup	0

#	Name	Amount	Points
20	Celery	1 cup (2 oz.) or 2 stalks	0
21	Chicory (curly endive)	1 cup or 6 oz.	0
22	Coconut, cream of	1/4 cup (2 fl. oz.)	5
23	Coconut, shredded	1 tsp.	0
24	Cranberries, dried	1/4 cup (1 1/2 oz.)	2
25	Cranberries, fresh	1 cup (4 oz.)	1
26	Cucumber	1 cup, 1 medium, or 4 oz.	0
27	Daikon	1 cup	0
28	Eggplant, cooked	1 cup (3 oz.)	0
29	Endive, Belgain (French)	1 cup (2 oz.)	0
30	Escarole	1 cup	0
31	Fiddlefern (fiddlehead greens)	1 cup	0
32	Gherkins, fresh	1 cup or 1 medium	0
33	Gourd, white, flowered	1 cup	0

#	Name	Amount	Points
34	Greens (beet, chard, collard, dandelion, kale, mustard, turnip), cooked	1 cup	0
35	Hearts of palm (palmetto)	1 cup (7 oz.)	0
36	Jerusalem artichokes (sunchokes)	1 cup (5 oz.)	0
37	Jicama (yam bean root, chop suey root, Chinese yam)	1 cup or 4 oz.	0
38	Kohlrabi, cooked or uncooked	1 cup or 2 medium	0
39	Ladyfingers, store-bought	1 large or 2 small (1/2 oz.)	1
40	Lamb's quarters, cooked	1 cup	1
41	Leeks, cooked or uncooked	1 cup or 2oz.	0
42	Lemon	1	0
43	Lettuce, any type	1 cup	0
44	Lotus root, cooked	1 cup or 16 slices	1
45	Mushrooms	1 cup	0
46	Mushrooms, breaded, frozen (prepared without fat)	7 (3 oz.)	3

#	Name	Amount	Points
47	Mushrooms, dried	1 cup reconstituted, 4 large, or 16 small	0
48	Mushrooms, marinated	1/2 cup	4
49	Mushrooms, stuffed	4	3
50	Okra, breaded, frozen (prepared without fat)	3/4 cup or 18 (3 oz.)	2
51	Okra, cooked	1 cup	0
52	Okra, fried	1 cup	8
53	Olive spread, store-bought	1 tbsp. (1/2 oz.)	2
54	Olives	10 small or 6 large (1 oz.)	1
55	Onion rings, fast food	1 medium serving(8-9 onion rings)	10
56	Onion rings, fried	4 (each 4" diameter) or 3 oz.	6
57	Onion rings, frozen (prepared without fat)	10 large rings(3-4" diameter)	7

#	Name	Amount	Points
58	Onion, blooming, battered and fried	1/4 (16" diameter)	6
59	Onions, cooked	1 cup	1
60	Onions, uncooked	1 cup	0
61	Parsnips, cooked or uncooked	1 cup or 6 oz.	1
62	Peas, dry, black-eyed	1/3 cup or 2 oz. cooked or 3/4 oz. uncooked	1
63	Peas, dry, split	1/3 cup or 2 oz. cooked or 3/4 oz. uncooked	1
64	Peas, green, cooked or uncooked	1 cup or 6 oz.	1
65	Pimientos, canned	1 cup, 6 whole, or 8 oz.	0
66	Plantain	1 cup (6 oz.)	3
67	Potato skins, frozen	2 (4 oz.)	5
68	Potato, baked, stuffed with bacon and cheese	1	8
69	Potato, baked, stuffed with bacon and cheese, fast food	1	13

#	Name	Amount	Points
70	Potato, baked, stuffed with vegetables and cheese	1	5
71	Potato, baked, stuffed with vegetables and cheese, fast food	1	10
72	Potato, baked, with sour cream and chives, fast food	1	8
73	Potato, stuffed with cheese, frozen	1 (5 1/2 oz.)	4
74	Potato, stuffed with sour cream and chives	1 (5 1/2 oz.)	4
75	Potato, sweet	1 large (8 oz. cooked or 10 oz. uncooked) or 1cup	3
76	Potato, white	1 large (8 oz. cooked or 10 oz. uncooked) or 1 cup	3
77	Pumpkin	1 cup	0
78	Pumpkin leaves	1 cup	0
79	Radish, white (Oriental, Daikon)	1 cup	0
80	Radishes	1 cup	0

#	Name	Amount	Points
81	Rhubarb, cooked, with sugar	1 cup	5
82	Rhubarb, uncooked, diced	1 cup	0
83	Rutabaga	1 cup	0
84	Salsify (oyster plant)	1 cup	0
85	Sauerkraut	1 cup (8 oz.)	0
86	Scallions (green onions)	1 cup or 16 medium (3 oz.)	0
87	Shallots	1 cup or 6 oz.	0
88	Snow peas (Chinese pea pods)	1 cup (4 oz.)	0
89	Squash leaves	1 cup	0
90	Squash, summer (caserta, chayote [pipinola, pattypan] , cocozelle, mirleton, scallop [cymling, pattypan] , vegetable marrow, yellow [crookneck, straightneck])	1 cup or 6 oz. cooked	0
91	Squash, winter(acorn [table queen] , banana, buttercup, butternut, calabaza, cushaw, Des Moines, dumpling, golden nugget, hubbard, peppercorn)	1 cup or 7 oz. cooked	1

#	Name	Amount	Points
92	Sugar snap peas, cooked	1 cup	0
93	Sweet potato leaves	1 cup	0
94	Sweet potatoes in syrup, canned	1 cup (9 oz.)	4
95	Sweet potatoes, candied	1/2 cup	3
96	Tamarinds	10 (2 oz.)	1
97	Tapioca	1 tsp. uncooked	0
98	Taro leaves	1 cup	0
99	Tomato and mozzarella salad	1 large tomato with 2 1/4 oz. cheese	10
100	Tomato, dried (not packed in oil)	4 halves (1/2 oz.)	0
101	Tomato, regular, fresh	1 cup or 1 medium (4 oz.)	0
102	Tomatoes, canned, all varities, packed in their own juice or tomato puree	1 cup (8 oz.)	0
103	Tomatoes, cherry	12 (4 oz.)	0
104	Tomatoes, plum	2 large or 4 small (about 4 oz.)	0

#	Name	Amount	Points
105	Tomatoes, stewed	1 cup (9 oz.)	0
106	Turnips, cooked	1 cup (6 oz.)	0
107	Vegetables, creamed (except creamed corn)	1 cup	10
108	Vegetables, fried	1 cup	6
109	Vegetables, in sauce, frozen	1 cup	1
110	Vegetables, mixed, drained	1/2 cup	0
111	Vegetables, packed in oil, drained	1 cup	3
112	Vegetables, pot roasted with pan drippings	1 cup	3
113	Vegetables, sauteed	1 cup	6
114	Water chestnuts	1 cup (4 1/2 oz.)	1
115	Watercress	1 cup (1 oz.)	0
116	Wax gourd (Chinese winter melon)	1 cup	1
117	Yams, cooked	1 large (8 oz.)or 1 cup	3
118	Zucchini, cooked or uncooked	1 cup	0

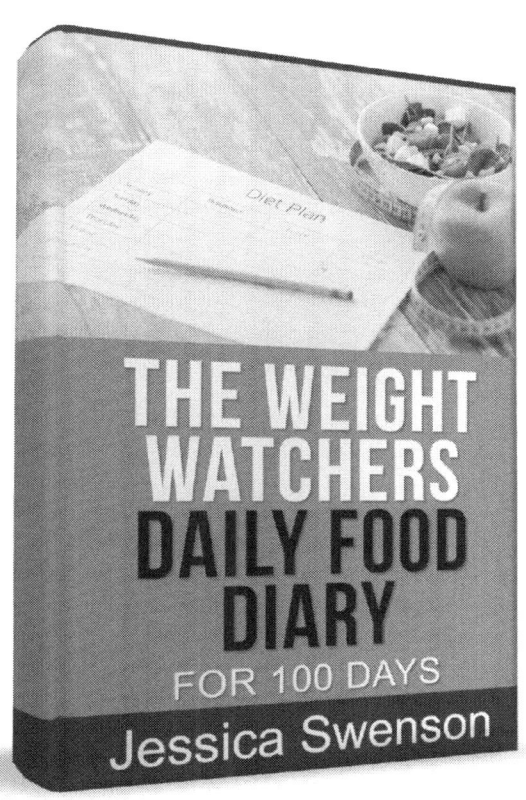

The Weight Watchers points system was designed to allow you to eat the sort of foods you like, but in measured quantities and within a certain food budget. Additional weekly points are also allocated and you can increase them when you exercise too, which is a great incentive. You can keep up to date with what you eat and the points you have remaining, meaning that you will always keep on top of your calorie intake.

And with this daily food dairy for 100 days, **The Weight Watchers Daily Food Diary,** is the ultimate weapon in your fight against obesity.

https://www.amazon.com/dp/1520828179

Made in the USA
Middletown, DE
22 March 2017